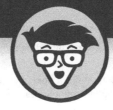

DBT
Workbook

by Gillian Galen, PsyD and Blaise Aguirre, MD

FOREWORD BY Mika Brzezinski

Co-host MSNBC's *Morning Joe* and founder of *Know Your Value*

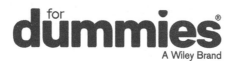

DBT Workbook For Dummies®

Published by: **John Wiley & Sons, Inc.**, 111 River Street, Hoboken, NJ 07030-5774, www.wiley.com

For general information on our other products and services, please contact our Customer Care Department within the U.S. at 877-762-2974, outside the U.S. at 317-572-3993, or fax 317-572-4002. For technical support, please visit https://hub.wiley.com/community/support/dummies.

Wiley publishes in a variety of print and electronic formats and by print-on-demand. Some material included with standard print versions of this book may not be included in e-books or in print-on-demand. If this book refers to media that is not included in the version you purchased, you may download this material at http://booksupport.wiley.com. For more information about Wiley products, visit www.wiley.com.

Library of Congress Control Number is available from the publisher.

ISBN 978-1-394-26308-0 (pbk); ISBN 978-1-394-26310-3 (ebk); ISBN 978-1-394-26309-7 (ebk)

SKY10077856_061924

Contents at a Glance

Foreword xi

Introduction 1

Part 1: Getting Started with DIY DBT 5
CHAPTER 1: Beginning Your DBT Journey 7
CHAPTER 2: Digging into the Benefits of DBT 27

Part 2: Preparing Yourself for Skillful Living 41
CHAPTER 3: Setting a Commitment to DBT 43
CHAPTER 4: Being Intentional 69
CHAPTER 5: The Principles of Behavior 95

Part 3: Practicing DBT 107
CHAPTER 6: Mindfulness 109
CHAPTER 7: Emotion Regulation 133
CHAPTER 8: Interpersonal Effectiveness 153
CHAPTER 9: Distress Tolerance 179
CHAPTER 10: Walking the Middle Path 203
CHAPTER 11: Digging into Dialectics 221

Part 4: It Doesn't End Here: Living a DBT Lifestyle 243
CHAPTER 12: Living a Life without Mood-Dependent Behaviors 245
CHAPTER 13: Focusing on Future Self 259

Part 5: The Part of Tens 283
CHAPTER 14: Ten Tips for a Skillful Life 285
CHAPTER 15: Ten Ways to Overcome Obstacles 297
CHAPTER 16: Ten Ways to Self-Validate 301

Index 309

Contents at a Glance

Table of Contents

FOREWORD xi

INTRODUCTION 1
    About This Book. 1
    Foolish Assumptions 2
    Icons Used in This Book 2
    Beyond the Book 3
    Where to Go from Here 3

PART 1: GETTING STARTED WITH DIY DBT 5

CHAPTER 1: **Beginning Your DBT Journey** 7
    The Origins of DBT 8
    Deconstructing Dialectics 14
        Searching for multiple truths in any situation 16
        DBT assumptions 19
        Assumptions about treatment 20
        DBT principles and protocols 21
    Modes of Therapy and Their Functions 23
        Therapy must tap into a person's existing capabilities 23
        Therapy must encourage a person's motivation to change 24
        A person's new capabilities must be relevant to all environments 25
        Therapy should enhance the therapist's motivation to treat people. 25
        Therapy should structure the environment so that treatment can happen. . . . 25
    Components of DBT 25

CHAPTER 2: **Digging into the Benefits of DBT** 27
    Unmanageable Emotions 28
        Born that way 28
        A deeper dive into emotional dysregulation 28
    Unrestrained Behaviors 31
    Disrupted Relationships 33
    Confused Cognitions 36
    An Unstable Self 38
        The impact of an unstable self 38
        What is identity? 38
    The Dysregulation Cycle 40

PART 2: PREPARING YOURSELF FOR SKILLFUL LIVING 41

CHAPTER 3: **Setting a Commitment to DBT** 43
    Pinpointing Your Problems 43
        Your perspective matters 44
        Are you solving the right problem? 44
        Sources of suffering 44

        Accurately defining the problem 46

        Being behaviorally specific 49

    Does Every Problem Need a Solution? 53

    Identifying Your Goals 55

        Short-term goals 57

        Long-term goals 58

    Making a Commitment to Change 59

        The key to success 60

        Barriers to commitment 61

        Overcoming barriers 64

    Generating Hope/Cheerleading 67

CHAPTER 4: Being Intentional 69

    Moving Beyond Your First Reaction 69

        Taking a breath 70

        Observing an urge 71

        Why surf an urge? 71

        Learning to urge surf 72

        Sensing the space 72

        Letting go of attachment 76

        Letting go of toxic relationships 82

    Reacting with Intention 85

        Considering different perspectives 85

        Breaking free from rigid choices 87

CHAPTER 5: The Principles of Behavior 95

    Taking the First Step 95

    Understanding the Function of Behaviors 96

    Recognizing Reinforcers 98

        Positive and negative reinforcement 98

        Extinction 99

    Understanding Shaping 103

    Pivoting on Punishment 105

        Effective punishment 105

        Ineffective punishment 106

PART 3: PRACTICING DBT 107

CHAPTER 6: Mindfulness 109

    What Is Mindfulness and What Are Its Benefits? 110

    Understanding Your Own Mind 110

        DBT states of mind 111

        Mindfulness of current thoughts 116

        Working with your cognitive distortions 118

    Practicing Mindfulness 120

        The "what" skills 120

        The "how" skills 124

    Setting a Routine and Building Your Practice 130

CHAPTER 7: Emotion Regulation 133

What Is Emotion Regulation and What Are the Benefits? 133
Understanding and Identifying Your Emotions. 134
    Finding the function of emotions 134
    Primary and secondary emotions 134
    Justified and unjustified emotions. 139
Naming Your Emotions and Decreasing Emotional Suffering 139
    Reducing emotional vulnerability with ABC PLEASE. 140
    SUN WAVE NO NOT. 146
    Changing how you feel with opposite action. 148

CHAPTER 8: Interpersonal Effectiveness. 153

Understanding What Gets in the Way of Your Relationships 154
Mastering DEAR MAN Skills 155
The Art of Validation 160
    Building blocks of validation 161
    Validating when you disagree 165
Communicating with GIVE Skills 167
Staying True to Yourself with FAST Skills 169
Combining GIVE and FAST Skills 172
Managing Interpersonal Anger with THINK Skills 173

CHAPTER 9: Distress Tolerance 179

What Is Distress Tolerance? 179
Employing Crisis Survival Skills 180
    Distracting with ACCEPTS and IMPROVE 181
    Calming yourself with self-soothing 185
    Taking the edge off with TIPP. 187
    Slowing down with STOP 188
    Making wise decisions with pros and cons 190
Accepting Reality 193
    Practicing radical acceptance. 193
    Turning the mind. 196
    Understanding willingness and willfulness 197
Putting It All Together: Your Own Crisis Kit 199

CHAPTER 10: Walking the Middle Path 203

What Is the Middle Path? 203
    Dialectics vs compromises 204
    Letting go of either/or and welcoming both/and 205
Middle Path Dialectical Dilemmas. 208
    Fostering dependency and forcing autonomy 209
    Too loose and too strict 212
    Making light of problem behaviors and making too much of
    typical adolescent behaviors 215

CHAPTER 11: **Digging into Dialectics** 221

    Recognizing the Dialectical Dilemmas 221
        Emotional vulnerability vs self-invalidation 222
        Active passivity vs apparent competence 222
        Unrelenting crisis vs inhibited grieving. 223
    Working Through Your Dialectical Dilemmas 225
        Dealing with emotional vulnerability 225
        Dealing with self-invalidation. 226
        Dealing with active passivity. 228
        Dealing with apparent competence 230
        Dealing with unrelenting crises 232
        Dealing with inhibited grieving 235
    Embracing the Paradox. 238

PART 4: IT DOESN'T END HERE: LIVING A DBT LIFESTYLE 243

CHAPTER 12: **Living a Life without Mood-Dependent Behaviors** 245

    Using DBT Skills to Regulate Your Emotions 246
    Wisely Setting Goals 246
    Breaking Down the Steps 249
    Maintaining Motivation. 250
    Observing Obstacles 254
    Eliminating Emotional Decision Making 255

CHAPTER 13: **Focusing on Future Self** 259

    Identifying the Person You Want to Be. 259
    Benefits of Connecting with Your Future Self 260
        What about your former self? 262
        Avoiding the future self traps. 264
    Recognizing Present-Self Behaviors 266
        Defining risky behaviors 266
        Why do people engage in risky behaviors? .274
    Aligning Your Present and Future Self 276

PART 5: THE PART OF TENS 283

CHAPTER 14: **Ten Tips for a Skillful Life** 285

    Periodically Review Your Short- and Long-Term Goals 285
    Never Stop Learning 288
    Practice Wholistic Health 288
        Regular exercise. 289
        Balanced diet 289
        Good sleeping habits. 290
    Limit Drugs and Alcohol 291
    Limit News and Social Media 291
    Be Accountable to Others. 292
    Accumulate Positives. 293
    Build Mastery 294
    Use the Coping Ahead Skill. 295
    Practice Flexibility 296

CHAPTER 15: **Ten Ways to Overcome Obstacles** 297

    Anticipate Obstacles When You Can. 297

    Validate the Emotions that Show Up 298

    Remember to Breathe 298

    Keep Your Goal in Mind 298

    Practice Effectiveness 298

    Understand the Problem 299

    Engage in Problem Solving. 299

    Ask for Help If You Need It 299

    Pivot If You Need To 300

    Use Encouragement to Stay in the Process. 300

CHAPTER 16: **Ten Ways to Self-Validate**. 301

    The Benefits of Self-Validation. 301

    Ten Steps to Validation 302

INDEX 309

Foreword

Dialectical Behavioral Therapy (DBT) has changed my life. Dr. Gillian Galen and Dr. Blaise Aguirre are on the forefront of a movement started by Dr. Marsha Linehan, one that had a far greater impact on my life than I would have ever imagined. What I have gained from DBT is almost impossible to condense into this short foreword, but it's worth trying.

Despite being blessed throughout my life in so many ways, chapters of my life have been more difficult than they needed to be because of avoidance, emotional dysregulation, and the inability to move past my own failings. This has led to fractured relationships, mental illness, and suffering for myself and my loved ones. I turned to DBT as the latest of several failed efforts to "fix" my relationships and myself. That journey, which proved to be more life-changing than I could have ever imagined, led me to the doorsteps of Drs. Galen and Aguirre.

As the cohost of "Morning Joe" and the creator of the women's empowerment platform "KNOW YOUR VALUE," I've had the opportunity to meet world leaders, as well as titans in all areas of business, arts, politics, and foreign policy. I have met people on the front lines of conflict resolution, peacemaking, diplomacy, geo-strategic negotiation, and relations around the world. In every aspect of conflict, discrimination, inequality, and even war, I am certain that DBT could dramatically improve and repair turbulence and upheaval. From peace in the Middle East, to managing NATO and Russian aggression, to the dangerous political divisions within the United States, if DBT were the norm, the question would not be how to solve these struggles, but rather whether these struggles even existed in the first place.

Division, anger, hatred, violence, and intolerance all come from a lack of acceptance, avoidance, and an inability to regulate emotions. DBT addresses all of these struggles. That is why this workbook can effectively be utilized by schools, colleges, businesses, and even governments around the world.

DBT works—in fact, the skills are so effective that one can move from a time in their life where they are diagnosed as "ill" and miserably depressed, to someone who experiences joy and a sense of steadiness and confidence. Fulfilled and *validated*. Through "KNOW YOUR VALUE," I teach women how to negotiate for raises and how to get "value back" in every relationship. Every tenant of DBT has made my message more effective and easier to teach. Learning skills like validation, radical acceptance, mindfulness, and, most importantly for me, emotion regulation—that's the value of DBT. Make no mistake: DBT takes consistent work. At the same time, this workbook makes it doable. *DBT Workbook for Dummies* walks you through the skills. With repetition, these skills can become second nature, and your life will start to get better and better every day. For me, the sun came up on all my relationships, and most importantly with the people I love—my family. These skills can save your relationships too, and the world.

—Mika Brzezinski, American talk show host, political commentator, and author

Introduction

I
f you recall from our first book, *DBT for Dummies,* dialectical behavior therapy (DBT) is a powerful evidence-based treatment developed by Dr. Marsha M. Linehan to help people navigate lives filled with emotional chaos and turbulent relationships. It combines elements of cognitive behavioral therapy (CBT) and change techniques with mindfulness and acceptance practices. By combining mind and body, DBT offers a more holistic approach to addressing mental health suffering.

This workbook was developed as a companion to *DBT for Dummies* and is designed to be a personal guide as you work toward a life worth living. Your journey will include practices that will reduce your emotional reactivity, increase mindful awareness, help you build more enduring and fulfilling relationships, and create an improved ability to tolerate difficult moments. If you read *DBT for Dummies,* you will be familiar with the therapy, and this book will help you deepen your understanding and practice, but even if you are new to the concepts of DBT, this workbook is here to support you every step of the way.

As you embark on this journey, remember that change is a process, and each small step you take brings you closer to your goals. This workbook is not just about completing exercises; it is about integrating these skills into your daily life, fostering a deeper sense of self-awareness and resilience. The book provides tips, reminders, and cross references as a way to interconnect the various skills into a toolbox of abilities.

About This Book

Within these pages, you will find a series of exercises, activities, and reflections carefully crafted to prompt the practice, strengthening, and generalization of the core DBT skills. From learning effective ways to manage intense emotions to improving effectiveness in relationships, each chapter is designed to build on the last, creating a solid foundation for your personal growth.

This book is meant to be written in; additional worksheets and practices are available online. Because these skills are meant to be practiced and integrated into your life, consider identifying worksheets that you may want to have on hand to help you practice certain skills throughout the day or week. One of the assumptions of DBT skills training is that DBT skills should be learned and generalized in all important contexts of your life. Our hope is that this workbook will be your guide.

You can use this workbook on your own, in individual therapy, and in your DBT skills group. Know that you are not alone; because of the power of DBT, millions of people worldwide are using the approach to create meaningful, fulfilling lives — ones with less suffering and more empowerment and self-agency. We hope this guide will be as helpful to them as it is to you.

Set aside some time for yourself, you deserve it! Take a deep breath, stretch your body, and let us join you on your journey to a more skillful and fulfilled you, with this workbook as your roadmap. You've got this!

Foolish Assumptions

As DBT therapists, we make few assumptions about you! You are reading this book to continue your quest to learn DBT and integrate these skills into your life. You may have some basic understanding of DBT, or this may be the first step to a more skillful life. We will guide you on this journey, and you must make the commitment to practice the skills. If you practice these skills, the way you live and experience your life will begin to change.

We recognize that no book is a substitute for expert therapy, and we assume that anyone who needs help will seek it out. We also assume that readers who are suffering may find these skills challenging and find change overwhelming, and we remain committed to acting as your guide and a place to come back to at any time. Finally, as all DBT therapists do, we assume that at any given moment, we are all doing the best we can, *and* we can always do better, try harder, and be more motivated to change!

Icons Used in This Book

Throughout this book, icons in the margins alert you to important types of information:

REMEMBER

This icon marks particularly noteworthy information that you might record or write down so you can refer to it later.

PRACTICE

This icon tells you it's time to roll up your sleeves and get to work! It denotes a worksheet, form, or exercise for you to fill out.

EXAMPLE

This icon points to specific examples that show you the way through worksheets or exercises. Examples are fictional composites that represent accurate struggles, but they're not real people.

WARNING

This icon appears when you need to take care; you may need professional help or should be on the lookout for possible trouble.

TIP

This icon alerts you to especially useful insights and explanations.

Beyond the Book

Throughout the book there are worksheets that you may want to complete more than once. Go to www.dummies.com/go/dbtworkbookfd to download blank versions that you can print and use.

In addition, there's a cheat sheet with tips and information about anxiety and depression. To access this online cheat sheet, go to www.dummies.com and then type "Dialectical Behavior Therapy For Dummies Cheat Sheet" in the search box.

Where to Go from Here

DBT Workbook For Dummies can help you deal with emotional chaos and turbulent relationships in your life. It's pragmatic, concrete, and goes straight to the point. As such, this workbook doesn't devote a lot of text to lengthy explanations or embellishments of basic concepts, so you may want to find out more about specific types of therapy and alternative treatments elsewhere. For that purpose, consider reading one or both of the companion books: *DBT For Dummies* (Wiley), *Depression For Dummies* (Wiley), and *Anxiety For Dummies* (Wiley).

1
Getting Started with DIY DBT

Chapter **1**

Beginning Your DBT Journey

For people all over the world, these past several years of unrest, divisiveness, fear, and uncertainty have increased stress significantly. Stress often precedes the emergence of emotional disorders, especially anxiety and depression. In the United States, recent surveys suggest that about 40 percent of the adult population suffers from notable symptoms of anxiety or depression. The rates of anxiety and depression among adolescents have also risen dramatically due to disruptions in their lives during these tumultuous times.

TIP

This workbook is designed to help with troubling emotions. It isn't meant to be a comprehensive review of emotional disorders. Many people choose to use this book along with professional counseling or therapy, and some use it on their own. If you want more information and an in-depth discussion of DBT, take a look at *DBT For Dummies.* If you want more about anxiety or depression, take a look at the latest editions of *Anxiety For Dummies* or *Depression For Dummies.*

WARNING

If your symptoms are numerous and severe or your life seems out of control, you should consult your primary care provider or a mental health professional. These worksheets aren't meant to replace trained mental health professionals — they're the only people who can really diagnose your problem.

The Origins of DBT

Dialectical Behavior Theory (DBT) was initially developed by Dr. Marsha Linehan PhD, a psychologist at the University of Washington. Her motivation was to help adult women with a condition known as Borderline Personality Disorder (BPD). BPD is characterized by a person having intense and painful mood swings, difficulties in intimate and close relationships, negative ways of thinking about oneself, self-destructive behavior, and suicidal behavior. For many people with BPD, this confluence of symptoms paired with the reality of the risk of suicide makes it one of the most difficult mental health conditions to treat. In fact, before DBT, BPD was considered a uniquely difficult psychiatric condition to treat and contributed to stigma about BPD.

What Dr. Linehan realized was that certain conditions and disorders such as borderline personality disorder (BPD) were characterized primarily by emotion dysregulation. In other words, some people had difficulty controlling their emotions and emotional expressions.

She hypothesized that these difficulties arose from the transaction between an individual's biological and genetic makeup and specific environmental factors, and she called her theory the *biosocial theory*. She noted that people with conditions like BPD had three prominent characteristics:

>> **Sensitivity:** They tended to be emotionally sensitive, which means that they experienced emotions more quickly and with more intensity than the average person in response to events that led to emotional expression.

>> **Reactivity:** Next, she noted that when emotions showed up, emotionally sensitive people had difficulty controlling their emotions and that this led to behavior dictated by their mood state. When emotionally sensitive people were in a good mood, they could get almost anything done, and when they were in a bad mood, they had a difficult time meeting the expectations of the moment. This type of behavior based on mood is termed mood-dependent behavior.

>> **Slow return to baseline:** And finally, she noted that when the emotionally sensitive person experienced these intense and heightened emotions, it took them longer than the average person to get back down to their emotional baseline.

REMEMBER Don't worry if the worksheets in this chapter reveal that you have a few symptoms of emotional dysregulation. Almost everyone has struggles; that's human. However, you should be concerned when these symptoms significantly interfere with your life. As mentioned in the Introduction, you can find blank versions of these worksheets online (at www.dummies.com/go/dbtworkbookfd) that you can print and use.

Take some time to go through Worksheet 1-1 and identify areas in which you have experienced intense emotional reactions.

PRACTICE

Worksheet 1-1   Emotional Reactivity

Do you recognize these characteristics in yourself? If you do, what are some examples of times when you have experienced this type of emotional response? In other words, give an example when you felt emotions quickly and more intensely, when you stayed emotionally upset for a long period of time, or when your emotional state changed. What did you do in those situations?

_____

_____

_____

_____

_____

Linehan recognized that there were five types of dysregulations that impacted people who had problems with managing their emotions. *Dysregulation* is a term used by therapists, and it means an inability to regulate or to control. Linehan noted that for emotionally sensitive people — and in particular those who did not have the skills to manage difficult situations and relationships in their lives — difficulties regulating the following five areas of daily experience persisted. These types of dysregulation are not one-time events, but rather are patterns of behavior that persist over time.

The five areas of dysregulation and areas for which DBT has been found to be most useful, are as follows:

» **Emotion dysregulation:** Emotion dysregulation is the inability to flexibly respond to and manage emotions in the context of difficult circumstances. Instead of a measured response, for people who struggle with emotion regulation, their responses are highly reactive. Typically, these moments of reactivity are brief, lasting at most a few hours. These emotions nevertheless feel overwhelming and out of control.

» **Interpersonal dysregulation:** Interpersonal dysregulation is the experience of being ineffective in close relationships. This can happen because of fear, whether the fear is real or imagined, that the person will be abandoned by those closest to them. In this context, the person with BPD will then become desperate to prevent the abandonment from occurring and will behave in ways to prevent the abandonment from happening. These desperate ways will often appear to be extreme to others.

Another hallmark of interpersonal dysregulation is that people with BPD tend to develop intense relationships with others, characterized by extremes. Sometimes they idealize the other person and other times they devalue the other person. These fluctuations can happen very quickly and leave the other person feeling bewildered.

>> **Sense-of-self dysregulation:** Sense-of-self-dysregulation is the experience of having very little consistency in one's identity. People with BPD can have a very difficult time defining themselves in terms of who they are as people, what their values are, and what their long-term goals and life-direction is. At times, they look to others and try to copy their behavior in order to fit in, but in many cases, this doesn't feel authentic. Another aspect of self-dysregulation is the experience of emptiness, which is an intense feeling of disconnectedness, aloneness, and feeling misunderstood.

>> **Cognitive dysregulation:** Cognitive dysregulation is characterized by relatively brief episodes of paranoid thinking or misperceiving reality, and this is particularly true during periods of stress. This means that when the person with BPD has high stress levels, they can begin to imagine that others are intentionally out to get them, even when there is no evidence that this is true. Then, at times when emotions are powerful and painful, and this is especially true if the person has experienced significant trauma, people with BPD can have episodes of *dissociation*, which is the feeling or thought that they are not real or that the rest of the world is not real. The physical seems to disconnect from the emotional self.

>> **Behavioral dysregulation:** Behavioral dysregulation is the manifestation of extreme, sometimes impulsive, and at times dangerous behaviors. These behaviors are often used as a way to deal with intense and unbearable emotions, and can include self-injurious behaviors, such as cutting and suicide attempts. Other such behaviors include eating behaviors such as binge eating, substance use as a way to self-medicate, dangerous sexual behaviors as a way to feel connected, and dangerous driving or excessive spending as a way to feel a rush of positive emotions. People often report that they feel out of control in these instances; like they don't have the ability to refrain from engaging in the behavior.

These five areas of dysregulation can often intertwine in very painful ways. For instance, emotional dysregulation can lead to cognitive, behavioral, and interpersonal dysregulation. Interpersonal dysregulation can lead to emotional dysregulation, and so on. For many, feeling like they don't have a stable sense of who they are can lead to feeling out of control. Use Worksheet 1-2 to reflect on the areas of dysregulation that you've experienced personally.

PRACTICE

Worksheet 1-2   Dysregulation

My experience of:

Emotional dysregulation

>> What are two or three examples of this?

>> What behaviors typically follow emotional dysregulation?

>> When does emotional dysregulation tend to occur (time of day, day of week, location)?

>> What tends to prompt emotional dysregulation (thoughts, other emotions, interactions with certain people?)

_____

_____

_____

_____

_____

_____

_____

_____

_____

Interpersonal dysregulation

>> What are two or three examples of this?

>> Are there particular people who tend to cause interpersonal dysregulation?

>> What behaviors typically follow interpersonal dysregulation (fights, yelling, avoidance)?

>> What tends to prompt interpersonal dysregulation (abandonment fears, disappointment, feeling judged)?

_____

_____

_____

_____

_____

_____

(continued)

Worksheet 1-2 *(continued)*

_____

_____

_____

Sense-of-self dysregulation

» What are two or three examples of this?

» What does sense-of-self dysregulation look like for you (constantly changing values, defining self by what others do, constantly changing aspirations and goals)?

» When does sense-of-self dysregulation tend to show up (applying for jobs, deciding on fashion, being asked to give an opinion on a politically charged topic)?

_____

_____

_____

_____

_____

_____

_____

Cognitive dysregulation

>> What are two or three examples of this (black and white thinking, certainty unsupported by facts, paranoia, dissociation)?

>> When does cognitive dysregulation tend to occur (under stress, with certain people, by painful memories)?

_____

_____

_____

_____

_____

_____

Behavioral dysregulation

>> What are two or three examples of this?

>> In what way are the behaviors potentially dangerous?

>> When does behavioral dysregulation tend to occur (time of day, day of week, location)?

>> What tends to prompt behavioral dysregulation (thoughts, interactions with certain people?)

_____

_____

_____

_____

_____

_____

Deconstructing Dialectics

The fundamental principle underlying the practice of DBT is the recognition and emphasis on a dialectical way of thinking. *Dialectics* is at the core of DBT and is the acknowledgment that seemingly opposing experiences — including thoughts, emotions, or behaviors — can coexist. Not only can they coexist, but even though they may seem opposite in perspective, they can both contain truths at their core.

EXAMPLE

Here is a simple example that highlights this. Imagine a game of basketball. One person roots for one team, and another person roots for the other team. At the end of the game, one person is happy and the other is sad. Both of those experiences are true, coexist, and make sense.

This applies to mental health as well. Within the DBT framework, reality consists of opposing forces and experiences in tension, not dissimilar from the two fans of opposing teams in the basketball game. When it comes to therapy, therapists often push their patients to change. However, because it can be difficult, the patient does not easily meet the idea of change. The therapist and the patient often have a common goal, and that is for the patient to be happier and more effective in their life, but one may be pulling and the other may be pushing. It may even feel like a tug-o-war when they seem to be pulling in opposite directions. A practical example of this is, for instance, a therapist pushing a socially anxious client to interact with a co-worker, and yet the client resists because their anxiety causes fear of interacting with others, which they resist out of fear.

Both the experience of wanting to change and of being scared of change — or preferring to stay with the life you know — can coexist, are true experiences, and are understandable from both the therapist's and the patient's points of view. It makes sense that the therapist wants the patient to change and that the patient is either resistant or afraid of change. For people with conditions like BPD, the prospect of facing the emotional turmoil and suffering that they often feel during therapy feels more painful than they are willing to bear.

DBT therapists have realized that it was by moving into a collaborative and accepting stance rather than one solely focused on trying to get their patients to change, that the possibility of change occurred. So, when the therapist balances and synthesizes both acceptance and change-focused strategies in a compassionate therapy, the patient experiences the freedom they need to heal. In many cases, prior to DBT, they have experienced the opposite. In the previous example, the DBT therapist with the socially anxious client would acknowledge the difficulty and fear and balance it with problem-solving to determine how to take steps toward the shared goal. They have either noted locking horns with their therapists who insisted that the patient had to change, or they experienced a passive though caring therapist, who simply listened and did not offer ideas that could help. Use Worksheet 1-3 to reflect on times when you've been caught in dialectical thinking.

PRACTICE

Worksheet 1-3   Dialectical Thinking

Have you ever locked horns or had moments in therapy when your therapist wanted you to change your behavior and you did not want to do what they asked?

Describe the situation:

_____

_____

_____

_____

1. What did your therapist want you to do? Can you make sense of why your therapist wanted you to do whatever they were asking?

_____

_____

_____

_____

2. Why did you not want to do it or find it difficult? How would you explain your struggle to make the change your therapist was asking to someone else? Does it make sense to you that it was difficult?

_____

_____

(continued)

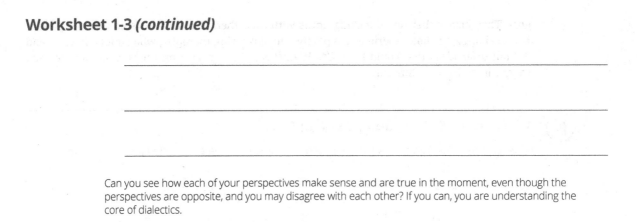

Can you see how each of your perspectives make sense and are true in the moment, even though the perspectives are opposite, and you may disagree with each other? If you can, you are understanding the core of dialectics.

In DBT, the therapist lets go of the need to be right and is open to the idea that there are other possibilities in the moment. Finally, in DBT, there is an emphasis on moving away from a rigid style of therapy and there is often a lot of movement, speed, and flow within a therapy session. This is achieved by the therapist using various strategies to increase or decrease the intensity, seriousness, lightness, or energy of the therapeutic interaction, and then assessing what works best for any one particular patient, rather than assuming that a single style works equally well for all patients.

The following sections delve more deeply into the dialectical process.

Searching for multiple truths in any situation

The core dialectic in DBT is that acceptance and change coexist. Here is an example. Imagine that you are stuck in very heavy traffic. You can't get out of the car, there are no nearby exits, and your mobile app tells you that you are at least an hour away from a meeting that you should have been at 30 minutes ago. What can you do? For some people, there could be rage, for others resignation, for others, an attempt to solve the problem a different way, for instance calling in to the meeting.

There are a few realities in the moment:

>> You are stuck in traffic.

>> There are no nearby exits to get out of the traffic.

>> You are 30 minutes late for a meeting.

>> You have a response to this situation.

Of course, more than anything, you would like the situation to change! You have two main options:

>> To accept the reality of the situation in the moment.

>> To reject the reality, or parts of the reality, of the situation in the moment.

So, if you decide that you are going to fully accept that this is the situation you are in, where does change come into the picture? A traffic jam can be aggravating, and especially if you are late for a meeting, it can lead to persistent suffering.

Another way to consider it is to say, "I cannot make the traffic be anything other than what it is, but I can change my reaction. I can learn to relax when I am in intolerable situations."

Imagine that you have an identical twin traveling in the car next to you, and you are both in the same traffic. Imagine that you were not accepting reality and fighting it all the way, feeling that it is unfair the traffic was so bad. What would your state of mind be? On the other hand, if your twin accepted that this is the reality in this moment and decides not to fight reality, but instead recognizes that the one thing that they can control is their state of mind and their reaction to the stressful situation, they would be in a far more relaxed state of mind. That represents change. Change and acceptance are occurring at the same moment. Research shows is that the more emotionally regulated a person is, the more capable they are of solving problems, and that the more dysregulated a person is, the fewer options come to mind.

REMEMBER

From a philosophical perspective, dialectics say that we have the *thesis* on one side, meaning one concept (the traffic is unbearable) and an *antithesis* on the other side, meaning an opposite concept (you can change your reaction to the traffic). Then comes what Dr. Linehan termed the *dialectical synthesis*, which is the integration of the two perspectives and that is, "I can be in a situation that I don't like, and yet accept it. By doing so, I can make the changes necessary to be more effective. Difficult moments become opportunities for me to learn to be more capable and skillful."

Worksheets 1–4 and 1–5 help you pinpoint coexisting opposites currently causing stress in your life and think of them in different ways.

Worksheet 1-4   Coping with Coexisting Opposites

PRACTICE

Think of a situation that you might be struggling with, such as a difficult relationship, struggles at work, or the urge to do behaviors that you know aren't healthy in the long run.

For example, if it is a relationship that you are struggling with, write down some facts about the relationship (the positives and negatives) and then reflect on what makes it difficult. Can a person who is supportive still have qualities that are unhelpful, and can a person who is less supportive still have qualities that are kind? Write down all the opposites.

TIP

Use the word AND rather than BUT. For instance, say your friend tends to be late for get-togethers. Saying "My friend is emotionally available AND at the same time unreliable when we make plans" says that both are true. Saying "My friend is emotionally available BUT unreliable when we make plans," tends to diminish the value of the friendship.

_____

_____

_____

_____

Worksheet 1-5   Depolarizing Experiences Using AND

What is the issue that tends to pull you into extremes?

Write down all the elements of the situation as clearly as you can, adding as many specifics as you can.

What are some of the benefits of the situation and what are some negatives? You can validate that the positives are positive and that the drawbacks are negative.

Next, is there a way that you can integrate the positives and negatives, using the word AND, to come up with a new way of seeing the situation?

_____

_____

_____

_____

_____

_____

_____

_____

_____

_____

_____

Here are some examples:

EXAMPLE   *I don't like the way my sister teases me AND she is always there for me.*

My coach is pushing me so hard that I am exhausted and want to quit AND her coaching is making me a better player.

It's painful that I didn't get invited to the party AND I am happy that I have the time to read my new book.

The point is that by simply focusing on the negative, you get stuck in suffering. There is always another side to a situation. Practicing thinking in this way can help you suffer less and see things more clearly.

REMEMBER

The bottom line: In DBT, dialectics is the practice of looking at the synthesis of thesis and antithesis. In doing so, the practice:

>> Acknowledges that change is the only constant in the universe, and that the process is continuous.

>> Acknowledges that all things are made of opposing forces.

>> Focuses on bringing together the most valuable parts of the opposing forces to form a new meaning, understanding, or solution in a given situation.

DBT assumptions

People are usually told to avoid making assumptions. Yet, every therapy operates with a certain set of basic assumptions. For instance, psychoanalytic therapy assumes that there is a *dynamic unconscious*, which is made up of the thoughts and feelings that are actively kept out of consciousness by the action of what Freud termed *defenses*. And like other therapies, DBT is no different. It operates with a certain set of clearly articulated assumptions. Having assumptions about patients and the treatment allows providers to agree and work together from a common place.

In DBT, therapists agree that they will see their patients and others while holding these assumptions in their mind. Assumptions about patients (and all of us):

>> People (all of us) are doing the best that they (and we) can.

>> People want to improve.

>> People need to do better, try harder, and be more motivated to change.

>> People must learn new behaviors, both in therapy and in the context of their day-to-day life.

>> People cannot fail in DBT.

>> People may not have caused all of their problems and they have to solve them anyway.

>> The lives of people who are suicidal are unbearable as they are currently being lived.

Many people, including therapists and loved ones, at first find it confusing to hold these assumptions in mind. When they see a patient or loved one behaving in self-destructive ways, they understandably ask, "How can I accept that my patient or loved one is doing the best they can?" The idea in DBT is that a person is doing the best they can, given their circumstances in that moment. Additionally, these assumptions help providers (and patients and others) start from a non-blaming and compassionate foundation. Use Worksheet 1-6 to challenge your own assumptions and learn to be kind and accepting of your efforts.

Worksheet 1-6 Assumptions

Think about this for yourself. Do you behave in the same way when you are hungry, tired, emotional, under the influence of substances, or sick? Can you accept that the best you can do when you are not feeling at your best is different from the best you can do when you are feeling beaten down?

Review the assumptions and see how they apply to you. Think about your vulnerability factors, your past treatments (if you have been in treatment before), and so on, and write down your reflections.

_____

_____

_____

_____

_____

_____

_____

Assumptions about treatment

In the same way that DBT has assumptions about patients, it also has certain assumptions about the treatment itself. All adherent DBT therapists review these assumptions and use them as guideposts to keep on track.

>> The most caring thing a therapist can do is help people change in ways that bring them closer to their own ultimate goals.

>> Clarity, precision, and compassion are of the utmost importance.

>> The treatment relationship is a real relationship between equals.

>> Principles of behavior are universal, affecting therapists no less than patients.

>> Treatment providers need support.

>> Treatment providers can fail, and they can fail in helping their patient even if they provide the best therapy.

Therapists recognize that they are human beings working with other human beings and that the influences that impact their patients also impacts them. They get sad, try their best, fail at times, and so on. And so, although therapists may have a greater ability to regulate their experience, they are just as human as you are!

DBT principles and protocols

Dialectical behavior therapy is based on certain principles and relies on certain protocols in its application. From a scientific perspective, the term *principle* means an idea or set of ideas based on scientific rules and laws that are generally accepted by scientists. At the heart of DBT philosophy sit the following principles:

>> **All things are interconnected:** From a DBT perspective, this assumes that a system must be analyzed as a whole and that all people are intimately related to and influenced by all the experiences and interactions that happen between them.

>> **Change is constant and inevitable:** From a DBT perspective, this implies that each of us and the environment are undergoing continuous transition. Because of this, DBT doesn't focus on maintaining a stable, consistent environment, but rather aims to help a person become more skillful in dealing with the inevitable change.

>> **Opposites can be integrated to get closer to the truth, also known at the *principle of polarity*:** This builds on the idea that not only is reality not static, but that it is made up of internal opposing forces. From a DBT perspective, this also means that within dysfunctions, there is also function, that within destruction, there is also birth, and that within chaos and distortion, there is accuracy.

What is interesting about these principles is that they are true when applied to DBT, and they also happen to be true in the context of physics and chemistry. At a practical and application level, the key principles in DBT are the principles of:

>> **Dialectics:** As explained earlier in this chapter, this is the idea that multiple and even opposing truths exist in any context.

>> **Behaviorism:** The idea that all behaviors are learned through interaction with the environment, and that behavior can be changed through the application of behavioral responses such as reinforcement, shaping, and punishment. Chapter 5 covers this principle fully.

>> **The biosocial theory:** The idea that emotional vulnerability and chronic environmental invalidation lead to dysfunction. DBT theorizes that problematic behaviors, emotions, thoughts, and relationships are caused by the interaction between a person's biological makeup and an invalidating environment. This theory is known as the *biosocial theory* or the *biosocial theory of emotional development*.

According to this theory, the interaction between your biology and your social environment leads to the development of your emotions and the behaviors that ensue. On the biological side, which is a product of genes and brain development, some people are more *emotionally* sensitive. The environmental element that most impacts the ability to regulate emotions is that of the pervasively invalidating environment. Invalidation is the experience of when private emotional experiences are ignored or punished or when the solution to dealing with painful emotions is oversimplified. This interaction over time can help explain why some people tend to struggle with significant and pervasive emotion dysregulation. This dysregulation can have a variety of serious consequences that include behavioral problems, out-of-control emotions, relationship issues, confusion about the self, and so on. People who benefit most from DBT often feel very validated by and relate to having the biosocial theory explained to them.

As an example, say you are an emotionally sensitive person (biology), and your private experience of a situation leads to a strong emotion — you are not invited to a party and you react by being extremely angry and sad at being left out. Let's then say that people in your environment tell you that you're making a big deal of the situation, or they say you should just call another friend, or tell you you shouldn't feel that way — these are all examples of being invalidated.

Interactions where you experience strong emotions that are invalidated over time are problematic because not only are these interactions emotionally painful, but further, they don't teach you how to manage the emotional experiences. Invalidation also increases disconnection in the relationship (not feeling understood), which can then increase painful emotions. Use Worksheet 1-7 to identify your own such experiences and emotions.

Worksheet 1-7   Validation and Invalidation

PRACTICE

Write about a situation that triggered an intense and painful emotional response.

_____

_____

_____

Next, write down the responses of other people who you felt were invalidating your feelings, meaning they said you were making a big deal of the situation, that you should just get over it, and so on. What were their responses, and how did you feel when they responded that way?

_____

_____

_____

_____

_____

_____

Did anyone respond in a validating way, acknowledging who you are and that how you felt was valid and understandable? What were these responses and how did they make you feel? (Chapter 8 goes much more into validation.)

_____

_____

_____

_____

_____

Hopefully, DBT in theory now makes sense, but what does it look like in practice? The next section covers that topic.

Modes of Therapy and Their Functions

In order to deliver DBT, Linehan identified certain modes or elements of the necessary treatment for it to be effective. These modes have specific functions that patients need in order to succeed.

She proposed that for DBT to be effective, the following criteria needs to be met. As you review these, see if they make sense and if they apply to you.

Therapy must tap into a person's existing capabilities

The first criterion is the idea that therapy must enhance a person's existing capabilities. This has two components:

>> **Any approach to therapy should recognize that all people have certain capabilities, ones that are effective and working in their life.** Many people who come for treatment don't believe that this is the case, feeling that they are good at nothing. This is often because the invalidating environment has led them to believe that their abilities and aspirations are of little value.

>> **Patients have to learn new and more adaptive skills in order to deal with life's challenges.**

Use Worksheet 1-8 to identify your own capabilities, as well as skills that you lack or need to work on.

Worksheet 1-8 Capabilities

PRACTICE

What are some of your existing abilities, ones that you are proud of, that make you feel competent, such as love of animals, compassion, artistic ability, and so on? Write them down.

_____

_____

_____

_____

Next, what are skills that you don't have that you need to learn, such as controlling your emotions, reducing the volatility in relationships, and so on? Write them down.

_____

_____

_____

_____

_____

Therapy must encourage a person's motivation to change

The second criterion is that therapy should enhance and maintain the person's motivation to change. Many times, people feel that they want to change and may even feel motivated to change, but then the effort seems to be too much and they give up.

A person's new capabilities must be relevant to all environments

The third criterion is that any therapy should ensure that a person's new capabilities are generalized to all relevant environments. What this means is that it is one thing to be a perfect and compliant patient in the therapist's office, but quite another to be skillful in your life. Is your therapy teaching you what to do in the relevant contexts in your life?

Therapy should enhance the therapist's motivation to treat people

The fourth criterion is that any therapy or approach should enhance the therapist's motivation to treat people who are struggling as well as enhance the therapist's capabilities through education and DBT practice. When therapists find that a patient has a complex set of symptoms, they can tend to feel bewildered and not know what to do. DBT therapy requires that DBT therapists be on a consultation team so that they can get help for their struggles, or as Linehan put it: "It is therapy for the therapists."

Therapy should structure the environment so that treatment can happen

The final criterion is that any therapy should structure the environment so that treatment can take place. In other words, are the conditions in place for therapy to be a viable option? What are the circumstances that are getting in the way of a person doing therapy, and can those environmental circumstances be dealt with? Does the person need help with transportation to therapy? Does the therapist need to speak to a school to advocate for a child to skip certain electives so they can come to therapy? Do you need a translator to help a person for whom English (or whatever language the therapy is being conducted in) is not their first language?

Components of DBT

In order to meet all these functions, comprehensive DBT has developed the following modes of therapy delivery: skills training group, individual treatment, DBT phone coaching, and a consultation team.

>> **Group:** The DBT skills training group is focused on enhancing a person's capabilities by teaching them behavioral skills. The group is run like a class, where the group leader teaches the skills and assigns homework for people to practice in their everyday lives. Typically, groups meet on a weekly basis for approximately two and a half hours. In standard outpatient DBT, it takes 24 weeks to complete the full skills curriculum.

>> **Individual therapy:** DBT individual therapy is focused on enhancing a person's motivation and helping apply the skills they have learned in group to the specific challenges and events in their lives. In the standard DBT model, individual therapy takes place once a week for approximately 60 minutes and runs concurrently with skills groups.

>> **Phone coaching:** DBT phone coaching is focused on helping people generalize the skills they have learned to problematic situations happening outside of individual or group therapy. Patients can call the person doing the skills coaching — who could be the individual therapist or another member of the team — between sessions to receive coaching ideas at the times when they need help the most.

>> **Consultation team:** The DBT therapist consultation team, therapy for the therapists, is there to support DBT therapists in their work with people who struggle with complex, difficult-to-treat disorders. The team helps therapists stay motivated and up-to-date so they can provide the best treatment possible. Teams typically meet once a week and are made up of anyone providing DBT therapy, whether individual or as group therapists.

TIP

Family therapy and case management can also be important in helping to structure the environment. Psychiatry for the monitoring of medication, when needed, is also helpful to enhance capabilities.

If you are looking for a DBT practitioner, it is reasonable to ask your potential therapist which modes of therapy they provide.

Chapter **2**

Digging into the Benefits of DBT

Chapter 1 explained that DBT works well for people struggling with five areas of dysregulation, *dysregulation* meaning an inability to effectively regulate or control thoughts and behaviors in these five areas. This chapter digs deeper into these five areas. It is key to remember that almost no one chooses to behave ineffectively, and they typically don't act effectively because they don't know how, or because the situation does not allow for effective skill use.

EXAMPLE

Here is an example of this concept. Let's say that you are visiting a friend from London, and they ask you to drive their car to the airport. You say that you cannot. Generally, the possibilities are twofold. The first is that you don't know how to drive, so driving the car would be impossible. The second possibility is that you do know how to drive, but because people in England drive on the left side of the road, you are worried that you don't have the skill to drive on the left, because you have driven on the right side of the road all your life.

As you learned in Chapter 1, the five areas of dysregulation are as follows:

» Emotion dysregulation

» Behavioral dysregulation

» Interpersonal dysregulation

» Cognitive dysregulation

» Sense-of-self dysregulation

Unmanageable Emotions

Emotion dysregulation refers to the inability to flexibly and effectively respond to and manage emotions, especially strong and painful ones. What is not included in this definition are the specific elements of emotional dysregulation. For some people, emotion dysregulation is a function of their emotion dysregulation. For others, it is because they are emotionally reactive and experience emotions intensely, and yet for others the environmental conditions make it difficult to use any emotion-regulation skills.

In actuality, many people experience all of these aspects, although between any two people how much each of these elements contribute to the difficulty in controlling emotions will vary.

Born that way

According to Marsha Linehan's biosocial theory, people with conditions like BPD (borderline personality disorder) are born being emotionally sensitive by temperament. This sensitivity leads some people to have a tendency to experience strong and painful emotions in many different situations and to seemingly trivial triggers, which in turn makes it difficult to learn adaptive emotion regulation strategies. Then, when they don't have adaptive and healthy coping skills, they might turn to unhealthy and maladaptive or even dangerous behaviors as ways to control their emotions. When unhealthy coping behaviors occur, these behaviors often lead to negative emotional experiences, which causes the cycle to begin again.

EXAMPLE

Here is an example of this cycle. 1) Imagine Jackie, a 28-year-old woman born emotionally sensitive, meaning that she feels things more quickly and more intensely and reacts strongly to seemingly trivial and insignificant provocations or triggers. 2) Because of this, it is difficult for her to learn coping skills. 3) She has a job as an administrator and overall has been doing well. Her boss calls her in to a meeting and tells her that because of her talents, he wants to promote her. However, before that happens, she has to improve her timeliness to meetings. Jackie only hears the criticism and concludes that her boss thinks she is a terrible employee who is never on time. It's all she can think about. As soon as she gets home, she opens a bottle of gin and has four shots in order to change how she feels. She wakes up the next day with a terrible hangover and realizes that she did not set her alarm and is going to be late for work. 4) She feels guilty and ashamed and the cycle begins again.

A deeper dive into emotional dysregulation

Enduring difficulty in regulating emotions is a manifestation of certain core elements:

>> **Emotional sensitivity:** Most people who struggle with emotion dysregulation are emotionally sensitive. Chapter 1 reviews this, and in this section, we want to define more clearly what we mean by emotional sensitivity. Emotion sensitivity is typically considered to be genetic and biological, meaning that a person is born emotionally sensitive.

Emotional sensitivity consists of a heightened emotional reaction to events that happen in the environment as well as events that happen in a person's mind. A heightened emotional reaction means one that appears to be above and beyond a typical emotional response. For instance, it is completely understandable that you would be upset if you weren't invited to some insignificant party that all your friends were invited to. If, on the other hand, you spent the next three days crying in bed, and it was all you could talk about, and it impacted your sleep and your relationships, that would be out of the regular range of responses.

However, emotional sensitivity is more than heightened reactivity. Emotionally sensitive people are also sensitive to the emotions of others. Some people are so sensitive to others' emotions that they can be feeling calm, walk into a room where people are sad or anxious, and then experience sadness or anxiety themselves. Keep in mind that not all emotionally sensitive people have BPD — their emotional sensitivity, when paired with the skills to manage it, can be very helpful, like for therapists, teachers, doctors or managing friendships.

>> **Enduring negative mood states:** Unfortunately, for people with conditions like BPD, emotional sensitivity is not a balanced experience. They experience more negative mood states — such as anger, anxiety, irritability, fear, and sadness — rather than positive mood states such as joy, surprise, and happiness, (although these more pleasant emotions can be dysregulated too). A consequence of this is that emotionally sensitive people tend to interpret situations negatively and are less accurate in identifying others' emotional states, for instance, frequently believing that others are angry at them or that others hate them.

However, the most important quality of the experience of negative mood is less about its absolute level and more about just how unstable the experience is. Meaning that you might be feeling miserable, and then experience a few moments of joy and feel some relief, only for the negative mood state to come back and intensify, at times, seemingly out of the blue. It is this reactivity that significantly influences the experience of negative mood states.

There is an apparent paradox in that people with BPD are — on the one hand — more sensitive to other people's emotions and — on the other hand — more likely to misinterpret others' emotions. The synthesis to these seemingly opposing ideas is that when emotionally regulated, they are very attuned to emotional changes in others. However, when they are emotionally dysregulated, their interpretation of others' emotions is inaccurate and tends to mirror their own emotion rather than reflect that there is something going on with the other person.

>> **Inadequate or maladaptive coping skills:** No suffering person chooses to be unskillful when they are in crisis. If they are not skillful, typically this is due to one of two reasons. The first is that they simply don't know what to do. Think of it this way. If you suddenly had to move to Italy and had never learned Italian, you wouldn't magically know how to speak Italian. Similarly, if you have never learned how to regulate your emotions, you can't suddenly know how.

The second reason is that even if you have some skills, the environment may be too complex or powerful so you find it difficult to use the skills you have. In the example of going to Italy, you may have some conversational Italian, but then going to a museum and having to follow a lecture on Renaissance art may be more than you can deal with. Similarly, you might be able to deal with some degree of sadness, but if you receive negative feedback at work, your friend cancels your dinner date, your dog is sick at home, and you are fighting with your parents, the level of distress may be more than you can handle. If you either don't have skills or the skills you have aren't enough to deal with the situation at hand, you might turn to quick but maladaptive solutions to deal with your emotions.

>> **Mood-dependent behavior:** We all have to get on in life, whether we are having a good day or not. If you wake up one morning, upset by an interaction that you had with a friend, you still have to go to work. For some people with very strong, painful, and difficult-to-control emotions, they can get almost anything done when they are in a good mood. But when they are in a bad mood, they aren't able to get anything done. This is known as *mood-dependent behavior*.

REMEMBER

The reason that some people have a hard time dealing with difficult emotions is because they never developed the skills to do so, or the situation is more complicated than the skills they have. It is rarely a choice that they don't want to be skillful, because if they are suffering, lack of skillful behavior makes them suffer more.

Use Worksheet 2-1 to reflect on whether and when you have problems dealing with your emotions. Then, in Worksheet 2-2, you'll reflect on the items you identify in this worksheet.

PRACTICE

Worksheet 2-1   Do I Have Problems Dealing with My Emotions?

Do you struggle with regulating your emotions? Before you begin to tackle a problem, it is key to know if something actually is a problem and then define the problem by identifying its specific elements. This worksheet identifies the elements and vulnerability factors of emotion dysregulation. Check the ones that apply to you.

❏ 1. I feel my emotions quicker than other people seem to feel them.

❏ 2. My emotions seem to last longer than they do for others.

❏ 3. Strong emotions seem to be prompted by relatively trivial issues.

❏ 4. When I feel my emotions, it takes longer for me to settle down.

❏ 5. When I am in a negative mood state, it feels nearly impossible to get anything done.

❏ 6. I tend to stay stuck in negative mood states.

❏ 7. I don't have the skills to manage very painful moods.

❏ 8. I do have the skills to manage most moods but at times, my life is so chaotic that my skills aren't enough.

❏ 9. I use behaviors that work very quickly but are not healthy to manage painful emotions.

PRACTICE

Worksheet 2-2   The Impact of Emotional Dysregulation on My Life

Now use this worksheet to reflect on the items you've checked. In the space provided, elaborate on the statements that apply to you and the impact that these experiences have had in various aspects of your life, such as friendships, work and academics, family relationships, and so on. Include all your thoughts, feelings, observations, and reactions.

_____

_____

_____

_____

_____

_____

_____

_____

_____

_____

Unrestrained Behaviors

When you are dealing with strong and painful emotions, you have the understandable desire to end your suffering. Some people aren't emotionally sensitive, so it is easy for them to "get over it." If only it were that easy. The previous section explained that emotional suffering is not a choice, but rather the consequence of either not having the skills to manage strong emotions, or having skills that are not adequate to deal with the situation.

In this context, many people turn to quick, often temporarily effective, and yet ultimately maladaptive, ways of coping. These include self-harm, drugs and alcohol, excessive spending, potentially harmful or unfulfilling sexual encounters, yelling and screaming at another person, unsafe driving, violence, and so on.

REMEMBER

If you are using potentially harmful behaviors to change how you are feeling, these behaviors are examples of behavioral dysregulation.

Behavioral dysregulation involves the enduring inability to block or stop maladaptive behavior, and, in turn, this can result in impaired functioning — as well as heightened levels of distress — in many areas of life. In disorders of behavioral dysregulation, people typically use more than one maladaptive behavior to attempt to regulate. For instance, people don't typically misuse just one substance. More common is the misuse of two or more. Similarly, they won't only use one category of maladaptive behavior, such as substance use. They will use other categories as well, such as dangerous sexual behavior, binge eating, spending, and self-injury.

Another element of these maladaptive behaviors is that there tends to be *behavior substitution*. For example, say that a person uses alcohol to self-regulate and that alcohol is now not available, or that they have decided to stop alcohol. It is common that a different behavior will take its place and that this behavioral substitution can start before the previous one has ended. For example, someone might start to binge eat just before they give up smoking.

Now, here is a key element to the concept of behavioral dysregulation. In the context of DBT, it is dysregulated behavior if the behavior functions to regulate painful emotions.

Let's say that you are at a party and watching two people have a drink. For one person, it is behavioral dysregulation and for the other it is not. How would you know the difference? As an outside observer, you would not know because the behavior can look identical. The key is *why* the person is drinking. If one is having a glass of wine because they enjoy wine, that is not dysregulation. If the other person is drinking because they are feeling embarrassed or upset about something, and they are drinking to change how they feel, that is problematic. Or, if you see someone eating a lot of food, if the person is bingeing to change how they feel, then that is behavioral dyscontrol. If, on the other hand, the person has just run a marathon, it would make sense that they are eating a lot of food.

Worksheet 2-3 is similar to Worksheet 2-1 in that you want to be clear about what constitutes behavioral dysregulation and what does not. This worksheet helps you identify the elements and functions of behavioral dysregulation. Use Worksheet 2-4 to reflect on and write about the items you identify.

PRACTICE

Worksheet 2-3   Do I Have Problems Controlling My Behaviors?

Do you struggle with regulating your behaviors? Be clear as to what constitutes behavioral dysregulation and what does not. This worksheet identifies the elements and functions of behavioral dysregulation. Check the ones that apply to you.

❏ 1. I use behaviors to control intense emotions.

❏ 2. The behaviors are potentially dangerous.

❏ 3. If one behavior is unavailable, I use a different one.

❏ 4. Behaviors include self-destructive ones like self-injury.

❏ 5. I use behaviors such as substance use to change my emotions rather than because I am using behaviors in a social context and because I enjoy the substance.

❏ 6. My maladaptive behaviors tend to help in the short run, but don't have lasting benefit.

❏ 7. My maladaptive behaviors tend to dull intense emotions, but then make me feel worse and cause more painful emotions later.

❏ 8. Even if I know healthier behavior to regulate my emotions, I feel that I need behaviors that will quickly change how I feel.

What makes a behavior problematic is its *function*. You might be enjoying a drink with friends because you enjoy the drink, and you enjoy their company. If, on the other hand, you are having the very same drink by yourself in your room in order to change how you feel, that is dysregulated behavior.

Worksheet 2-4   The Impact of Behavioral Dysregulation on My Life

PRACTICE Now use this worksheet to reflect on the items you've checked. In the space provided, elaborate on the behaviors that apply to you, and the impact that these behaviors have had on various aspects of your life, such as friendships, work and academics, family relationships, and so on. Include any beneficial aspects to the behaviors as well as the long-term emotional consequences of your behaviors.

_____

_____

_____

_____

_____

_____

_____

_____

Disrupted Relationships

Healthy relationships are a crucial part of happiness and individual growth. Close relationships, whether with friends, family, coworkers, or romantic partners, allow for the healthy expression of empathy, trust, effective communication, and interdependence. They are manifest by reasonable expectations of each other, mutual concern about the other person's welfare, and freedom to be who you are without the fear of judgment.

However, for some people who are emotionally sensitive and who experience emotional and behavioral dysregulation, the formation of healthy relationships can be complicated. You might want others to change their behaviors but find it difficult to change yours. Or, you might not like yourself and feel strongly that others won't like you either. Or, you may feel that if people really got to know you that they would leave you so you fear being abandoned.

When this kind of behavioral dysregulation happens, it can lead to significant interpersonal problems. People with BPD experience rapidly forming, and often rapidly dissolving, intense and unstable relationships. These relationships are characterized by intense fears of abandonment as well as swinging between idealizing others and then devaluing the very same people.

The interpersonal problems tend to be recurrent and repeated difficulties in relationships and in particular in the relationships to those who are closest. The theory is that people struggle in relationships because of early childhood experiences and insecurities, where they were uncertain as to their own sense of connectedness.

The behaviors that are most concerning tend to fall into two categories:

>> The first category defines behaviors that show up when a person feels abandoned. In the context of feeling abandoned, many people will go to great lengths to prevent the abandonment, and those behaviors occur whether the abandonment is real or imagined. A person may make repeated calls, send incessant texts, beg for reassurance, and so on, in order to know whether the person is going to leave them. The problem tends to be that these behaviors are often so off-putting to the other person that it becomes more than they can tolerate, and they end up leaving the person, even if that was not their original intention.

>> The second is that they might idealize a person one moment, imagining them to be the best person ever, and then devalue them the next, wondering what they ever saw in them. These swings are often driven by mood states and can be very confusing to the other person.

REMEMBER

Volatile relationships not only impact you, but the other person as well. Often, the very behaviors that you use to keep the person close can be more than the other person can tolerate and leads them to not want to be close to you.

Worksheet 2-5 helps you identify the elements of your problematic relationships and Worksheet 2-6 helps you reflect on the items you identify.

PRACTICE

Worksheet 2-5   Do I Have Problems in Close Relationships?

Do you struggle in your relationship with others? This worksheet identifies the elements found in problematic relationships. Check the ones that apply to you.

- ❑ 1. I get very close to people very quickly.
- ❑ 2. When I do get close, I feel that they are "the one" very soon after meeting them.
- ❑ 3. I tend to idealize people, even when they show me less than ideal qualities.
- ❑ 4. I tend to devalue people, even when they show me admirable qualities.
- ❑ 5. I fear that people are going to abandon me.

□ 6. When this happens, I become desperate.

□ 7. When I become desperate, I do anything to keep them.

□ 8. I need constant reassurance that others won't leave me.

□ 9. At times, I do dangerous things to see if people care about me.

Worksheet 2-6   The Impact of Interpersonal Dysregulation On My Life

PRACTICE Use this worksheet to reflect on the items you've checked. In the space provided, elaborate on the relationships you have and the impact of your behaviors on the relationships as well as the impact of others' behaviors on you.

_____

_____

_____

_____

_____

_____

_____

_____

Confused Cognitions

For all humans, when emotions get strong, thinking can get a bit disorganized (such as when someone has a big, stressful project and can't find their keys, which otherwise doesn't happen). For people with BPD, the emotions are bigger and the cognitive component is also much bigger.

Cognitive dysregulation is when you start to believe that everything that you think is real and start reacting to your thoughts as if they were real. This can manifest in the form of paranoia about the intention of others, as well as *dissociation*, which is a loss of touch with what is real and what is not. One can experience the following, which can then lead to emotional dysregulation:

>> *Catastrophizing* is the behavior of imagining or acting as if the only outcome is the worst possible outcome.

>> *Rumination* is the repeated thinking of, or dwelling on, a present situation or past memory.

>> *Avoidance* is the act of actively and intentionally staying away from any situation, memory, or people in order to prevent negative thoughts or consequences.

>> *Thought suppression* is the conscious attempt to stop thinking a specific thought.

Emotional dysregulation can also present as black-and-white, or all-or-nothing thinking. This type of thinking manifests in statements like "you always do abc," or "you never do xyz." Or, "if you don't love me 100% then that means you hate me," and so on.

Although these are some of the more common and researched cognitive struggles, there are other areas of thinking problems that many people with conditions like BPD experience. They often struggle with attention and concentration, tend to have short- and long-term memory problems, find it difficult to plan and know how to organize their day, and do not know how to effectively problem solve.

What can be particularly confusing, especially for those around them, is that the experience of some of these cognitive problems is not always evident to others. For instance, someone may feel that they have a terrible memory. In many circumstances, people who get psychological testing for memory problems show no deficits in memory at all. Or, people who feel that they can't plan their day are able to get back and forth to work or school without the organization being a problem. Often, the issue is less that their brains don't "work properly" as much as that strong emotions tend to impact the experience of thoughts and cognitive functions.

This can be true of almost anyone. Say you have a severe toothache. Your experience of ten minutes of an excruciating toothache will feel like an eternity, whereas your experience of ten minutes of your favorite activity will feel like a very short time. At times, events are retold less in a sequential order, and more in terms of their order of emotional importance. To others, it can appear as if you are lying, or omitting critical parts of the story. But for you, it is the way you remember events. Strong emotions also tend to impact the way that memory is stored and things are remembered. If you are studying for a test, you will find it far more difficult to remember what you studied if you are in severe emotional distress than if you are emotionally calm.

Thinking, planning, and remembering are often not impaired in people with strong emotions. It is more the case that strong emotions impact the way they think, plan, and remember. You will notice that, if you can bring down your level of emotional distress, your thinking, planning, and remembering will improve.

Use Worksheet 2-7 to identify the types of thought cognitive experiences that apply to you. Then use Worksheet 2-8 to reflect on the items you identify.

PRACTICE

Worksheet 2-7   Do I Have Problems in How I Think?

Do you struggle with your thinking? This worksheet identifies the types of thought cognitive experience that people with strong emotions experience. Check the ones that apply to you.

❏ **1.** I tend to think in black-and-white ways, especially when I am emotional.

❏ **2.** I tend to make all-or-nothing statements such as "you never," "I always," and so on.

❏ **3.** When I am under stress, I tend to think that people are talking about me.

❏ **4.** When I am under stress, I tend to believe that the world around me is not real.

❏ **5.** When I'm under stress, I have the experience of believing that I am not real.

❏ **6.** I have a hard time paying attention and concentrating, especially when I am feeling very emotional.

❏ **7.** I have a hard time remembering past experiences in a coherent timeline, and at times, people seem confused by how I tell stories.

❏ **8.** I have a difficult time planning my day because everything feels overwhelming to me, and I find it hard to know how to organize things.

PRACTICE

Worksheet 2-8   The Impact of Cognitive Dysregulation on My Life

Use this worksheet to reflect on the items you've checked. In the space provided, elaborate on how your thinking feels off in different aspects of your life and whether your thinking is particularly impacted by your emotional state.

_____

_____

_____

_____

_____

_____

An Unstable Self

Many people who come to DBT looking for help struggle with a distorted sense of self, a poor self-image, or tend to see themselves as fragmented, ashamed of who they are as people, and with no sense of direction or purpose. If you struggle similarly, you might notice that in an attempt to define yourself more clearly, you make sudden and even dramatic changes.

The impact of an unstable self

This can take the shape of changing your life goals, political and religious opinions, group of friends, appearance, or professional or academic aspirations. Sometimes, it is driven by the idea that if you don't have a sense of who you are, you can imitate people who seem to have a sense of who they are and, therefore, define yourself more clearly.

Your sense of self is closely tied to your identity, and when you struggle with a sense of who you are, you might experience yourself as fluctuating and inconsistent. This can feel particularly unsettling.

What is identity?

The concept of identity is the overall view of the way in which you see yourself. A stable sense of identity means that you see yourself today pretty much the way you saw yourself yesterday and the way that you imagine you will see yourself tomorrow. This also allows you to know when you have behaved in a way that is consistent with your value system and know when you have betrayed your values.

TIP

The elements of identity include your beliefs, opinions and attitudes, your perception of your abilities, your behaviors, and the way you act around the people in your life.

A strong sense of identity is critical for dealing with life's inevitable changes and challenges. For instance, if you know that you are a person who is drawn to compassionate people who have a sense of humor, who like animals and the outdoors, you will be very unlikely to spend time with a person who is into hunting animals and who wants others to admire them and gets angry when they don't. Now, if you don't have a strong identity or sense of self, you might fluctuate and feel that such a person is all you deserve and then agree that the way they are living is the way you should live because you feel that they are confident and you want to feel confident.

REMEMBER

An unstable sense of who you are is unsettling. Many people change their opinions over their lifetime, but if you have an unstable sense of self, it does not feel as if these changes are chosen or intentional. You might feel as if they overtake you and that you have to make changes in order to survive because you hope that those changes will anchor you in stability.

Worksheet 2-9 helps you identify the elements of a poor sense of self and unstable identity that may apply to you. Then use Worksheet 2-10 to reflect on the items you identify.

Worksheet 2-9　Do I Struggle with Knowing Who I Am and My Sense of Self?

PRACTICE

Do you struggle with a sense of who you are? This worksheet identifies the elements of a poor sense of self and unstable identity. Check the ones that apply to you.

❏　1.　I often question who I am.

❏　2.　My interests change quickly.

❏　3.　My political, religious, and societal beliefs change quickly.

❏　4.　I am not sure what my values are.

❏　5.　I become very interested in a professional career only for this to change, and I question what I am doing.

❏　6.　I tend to follow what my friends are doing — their interests and their fashions.

❏　7.　It unsettles me when people ask me what I am doing or what I want to do with my life.

❏　8.　I dread thinking that my different groups of friends will bump into each other when I am around because I act very differently with different groups.

❏　9.　I question my abilities and at times I am surprised that people think that I am good at things.

❏　10.　I sometimes feel empty, like there's a hole in how I think of myself.

Worksheet 2-10   The Impact of Self-Dysregulation on My Life

PRACTICE

Now use this worksheet to reflect on the items you've checked. In the space that follows, consider how your unstable sense of self has impacted your dreams of the future, life choices, and value system. Consider how this has impacted your career and academic interests, group of friends, and other affiliations.

_____

_____

_____

_____

_____

_____

_____

_____

_____

The Dysregulation Cycle

We have divided the five areas of dysregulation into discrete categories, and this is because DBT has different skillsets for each of the five areas. In reality, a person coming to DBT struggles with each of these five areas of dysregulation, and they interact with each other.

For instance, say you have a poor sense of self (self-dysregulation) and do not believe you are loveable. You become paranoid, convinced that your significant other is plotting to leave you (cognitive dysregulation). In this context, you start begging the other person not to leave you, telling them that they are the best person ever and that you cannot live without them. The behavior is confusing to the other person, and the relationship becomes increasingly volatile (interpersonal dysregulation). You become sad and angry that you are going to be abandoned, and you say hurtful things to them, which in turn leaves you feeling guilty and ashamed (emotional dysregulation) that you said hurtful things.

You struggle with these emotions and then use substances and self-injury (behavioral dysregulation) to reduce the amount of emotional suffering. Although you temporarily feel better, you then feel even worse that you resorted to those behaviors and imagine that people think you are a total failure and they hate you. You eventually feel that it is time to give up on the relationship you have and look for another relationship. The cycle begins again, and all the areas of dysregulation weave into a complex web of dysfunction. But fear not, because later chapters explain what you can do about each of these situations.

2

Preparing Yourself for Skillful Living

Setting a commitment to do something difficult by holding your long-term goals and values in mind

Moving from an automatic and habitual life to a more intentional one

Learning the principles of behaviorism, how these principles apply to all beings, and how you can use them to change your own and others behavior

Chapter 3

Setting a Commitment to DBT

C hapters 1 and 2 reviewed the types of problems that DBT works well on, and if you identify with some of the struggles, DBT might be the right treatment for you. It's one thing
to know that something is going to be helpful, but it is another thing entirely to make a
commitment to the work. This is true of many aspects of life. Many people know that exercising is a healthy activity, but simply knowing that doesn't mean that they will exercise.

As with any other therapy, people who seek out DBT therapy do so because they are struggling
in some way. However, it is not always clear exactly what the problem is, and in some cases,
part of the problem is not knowing what the problem is.

Pinpointing Your Problems

Many of us have had the experience of others telling us what our problem is. Usually, it is in
the shape of: "You know what your problem is," and then they go on to tell us the many ways
in which we are problematic. Often this is said when the other person is very upset. A variation
of this happens when a loved one accompanies a person to therapy and speaks for the patient,
saying something like, "Their problem is that they drink too much," or "They don't exercise
enough," and so on. In this case, it is likely that the loved one has great intentions and wants
to help.

Your perspective matters

A problem is most importantly a problem if it is a problem to you. If you have a glass of wine with dinner and your loved one thinks that any drinking is a problem, but you do not, and it's not causing you any difficulties in your life, you are not likely to commit to stopping. Of course, there are times when something that you don't think is problematic is actually problematic for a loved one, and then you have to consider what to do. The problem for you might not be what the other person says is the problem; however, the fact that you are in conflict with someone you love might be a problem.

EXAMPLE

For instance, say that you work long days, and you have to get up early for work. You go to bed early each evening. Your loved one tells you that it is problematic that you are going to bed early because it means that you can't do things like watch a movie, go out dancing, or even just talk. There is nothing inherently wrong with going to bed early and, in fact, if you want to be productive at work, you need a good night's rest. On the other hand, your partner feels excluded and feels that your going to bed early is preventing normal relationship activities. For you, going to bed early is a solution. For your partner, it is a problem. For your partner, your staying up late would be a solution, but for you, it would be a problem.

REMEMBER

Key to any type of therapy is knowing if there is a problem, identifying the problem, understanding how the problem impacts your life, and then determining what you can do about it.

This type of approach works well in many other situations where there is a problem. If your car is losing oil, going to the mechanic and saying, "I think that my car has a problem, because there was a pool of oil under it this morning, and when I started to drive, it made a strange noise. I am worried I won't be able to get to work and do other errands. Is there anything that can be done about this?"

Of course, life's problems are not always that clear or easy to solve, but the approach is similar.

Are you solving the right problem?

If you recall Jackie from Chapter 2, she became upset after her boss called her into a meeting and discussed her tardiness. Because of her emotional upset, she wanted the problem of being upset solved. So, she turned to alcohol, which was a solution in the short run, but made things worse in the long run. She was trying to solve the problem of her situation in the moment, but her solution was not effective and did not teach her what to do in a more general way.

Before delving more into why defining your problems is key, let's look at the sources that cause psychological problems.

Sources of suffering

Many different circumstances can cause the types of psychological suffering that lead to psychological problems. Here are the ones that most commonly lead people to look for DBT therapy:

>> **Childhood abuse, trauma, or neglect:** These three sources of adversity, and particularly in emotionally sensitive children, put people at risk for mental health problems and deficits in problem-solving skills.

>> **Loneliness:** When people are lonely or socially isolated, this can cause the type of despair that then leads to problematic behavior. This can be aggravated by bereavement when you lose someone who was a support and provided companionship.

>> **Social issues:** The stigmatization of mental illness, political, gender, or religious discrimination, and financial difficulties are all examples of this. These can be aggravated by difficulties in finding employment or loss of a job, or difficulty in finding housing.

>> **Chronic medical conditions:** Even if you have general mental wellness, chronic medical conditions can rob you of everyday experiences and joy to the point that it leads to mental health problems.

>> **Drug and alcohol misuse:** Sometimes, drugs and alcohol are used as a way to self-medicate, but in other situations, the misuse of drugs and alcohols are their own problem. Either way, whether cause or effect, they are often issues that need addressing.

Of course, there are many other things that happen in a life that can lead to suffering — events such as traumatic brain injury, domestic violence, and so on. However, these are the more common causes of suffering that lead people to DBT. Use Worksheet 3-1 to consider the causes of suffering in your own life.

PRACTICE

Worksheet 3-1   The Causes of Suffering in My Life

What are some of the events that have led you to suffer? List all of the causes in as much detail as possible. Then list the problematic behaviors associated with each cause. Use the blank pages in the back of the book if you need more space.

1. Cause of suffering and problematic behavior.

_____

_____

_____

_____

_____

2. Cause of suffering and problematic behavior.

_____

_____

(continued)

_____

_____

3. Cause of suffering and problematic behavior.

_____

_____

_____

_____

_____

_____

Accurately defining the problem

It might be obvious that you have a problem. Clearly, if you are suffering, something is wrong. But what exactly is the problem? In the context of psychology, one definition could be something that makes you suffer. Or it could be any obstacle that gets in the way of attaining a personal goal.

Chapter 1 highlighted that people who are in DBT typically struggle with emotional, behavioral, interpersonal, self, or cognitive dysregulation. These often interact with each other. However, it is important to identify what the problem actually is, because the clearer the definition, the easier it is to know what skill to use.

Think of it this way. Say your mom has a 20-pound box of tools, and she says that she has a problem, and could you bring her the tools? If she is not clear about the project she is working on, having to lug an entire box of tools around the house might be exhausting. If, on the other hand, she tells you that she is trying to hang a picture, you know what tools she needs, and you bring her a hammer and nail.

REMEMBER

Another important thing to remember. Just because something is a problem for someone else, does not mean that it is a problem for you. For instance, say that your best friend has a gluten allergy. It is a problem for them but not necessarily for you. This does not mean that you shouldn't be careful with cooking or restaurant choices when you are having dinner together, only that one person's problem is not another's.

Drilling down on the areas of focus for DBT, consider these questions:

>> If you struggle with emotions, is the problem that they are too intense? That you numb out? That they are too quick?

>> If you struggle with unhealthy behaviors, is it the types of behaviors? That the behaviors only last for a few minutes? That they lead to problems in other areas of your life?

>> If you struggle interpersonally, is it that you attach too quickly to people who end up hurting you? That you let people walk all over you? That you are a people pleaser? That you don't know how to set limits? That you don't let people get close for fear of getting hurt?

>> If you struggle with your sense of self, is it that you are constantly changing your values? Your job aspirations? Your groups of friends? The way you see yourself?

>> If you struggle with thoughts, is it that you are always thinking the worst of any situation? That you think in black-and-white or all-or-nothing ways? That you feel paranoid a lot of the time?

Use Worksheet 3-2 to consider the problem areas in your own life.

PRACTICE

Worksheet 3-2   The Problem Areas in My Life

What are the specific areas of your experience that are causing problems? Review the five areas listed in this section and define, as clearly and precisely as you can, which aspects within each of these areas are problematic for you. Also, if you can, identify why they are a problem.

1. Problems caused by my emotions.

    _____

    _____

    _____

    _____

    _____

(continued)

Worksheet 3-2 *(continued)*

2. Problems caused by my behaviors and problematic behaviors.

_____

_____

_____

_____

_____

3. Problems in relationships.

_____

_____

_____

_____

_____

4. Problems with my sense of self.

_____

_____

_____

_____

_____

5. Problems in the way that I think.

_____

_____

_____

_____

Being behaviorally specific

You have now identified the problem areas in your life. However, it is still important to be as clear and specific as possible. For instance, say the problem is that you feel overwhelmed, and you say so. Clearly, feeling overwhelmed is a problem; however, it neither tells the listener nor yourself what the actual problem is.

If, on the other hand, you say, "I have a big presentation tomorrow, I haven't walked the dog, and I haven't made supper. I am feeling as if there is too much to do right now," you are being clear and specific. That way, you and the listener have a better chance of figuring it out. For instance, your roommate might say that they will walk the dog and cook dinner because they've been wanting to try a new recipe.

Even if no one can help you immediately, breaking it down makes it easier to think of solutions. Maybe you normally walk your dog in the evening. Might you focus on your presentation and then walk the dog in the morning? Would you consider ordering a meal on an app? Is it time to break out the microwave meal that has been sitting in your freezer for the past two months?

Avoid vague language

There is another element to this and, unfortunately, it is a problem perpetuated by the mental health field itself: the use of vague language.

For instance, the following terms are often used in the field, but they are not clinical terms. Acting out, closure, denial, splitting, manipulative, gamey, attention-seeking, and so on. The reason these terms are problematic is that they are not precise and are interpretations by the observer. For instance, say an adolescent asks their father for $10, and the father says no. The adolescent then asks the mother, and the mother says yes. Someone might say that the adolescent is being manipulative, but if that is all the information we have, we don't have the complete story. Maybe the father does not have the money on him, and the mother does, maybe the father feels that the child needs to work for the money, and the mother does not feel that way.

Maybe the child was not very clear as to why they needed the money when asking their father but was more clear when asking their mother, or maybe the child wanted to pit the mother against the father. Without more information, we don't actually know their motive.

Avoid assigning intention

Being as behaviorally specific as possible takes the guesswork out of what is going on. What we mean by being behaviorally specific is that all people watching the same scene would say almost the same thing about what they saw. Say that a man was standing on a street corner with his right arm extended and his finger pointing. All we could say is that "a man is standing on a street corner with his right arm extended and his finger pointing." That is being behaviorally specific.

Unless we know otherwise, we cannot say that he is doing it for attention, that he is pointing at anything in particular, or anything else. In the absence of any other information, we cannot know his intention. People who come to DBT are often certain that they know the intentions of others, and yet unless those intentions are explicitly stated, we can never know. All we can see is behavior. Not intention.

One of the DBT consultation team agreements — and if you recall from *DBT For Dummies*, the *consultation team* is a group where therapists meet regularly to discuss their experience and ask for help when needed in the delivery of DBT — is the *phenomenological empathy agreement:*

> All things being equal, we agree to search for non-pejorative or phenomenologically empathic interpretations of our patients', our own, and each other's behavior. We agree to assume we and our patients are trying our best and want to improve. We agree to strive to see the world through our patients' eyes and through one another's eyes. We agree to practice a nonjudgmental stance with our patients and with one another.

So, central to DBT is the idea of not judging and not interpreting. If a therapist is going to interpret, they first describe behavior as behavior and then make an empathic interpretation if needed.

TIP

DBT asks that statements be behaviorally explicit. Describe what can you see, smell, hear, taste, and touch.

Instead of using words like manipulative, attention-seeking, and so on — words that are not behaviorally specific — describe what it is that you see. In doing so, you will realize that you might not know why somebody else is doing what they are doing, and they might not know why you are doing what you are doing.

EXAMPLE

For example, say the trash collector is coming and a mother shouts up the stairs and tells her son to take out the trash in time for the collection, before he goes to school. The son instead takes the dog for a walk. His father ends up taking out the trash. "He is so manipulative," says his mother to his father. "Do you see how he got out of it?"

What are the other possibilities?

>> Maybe the son didn't want to take out the trash and took the dog out knowing that his father would do it. Some would consider this manipulative.

>> Maybe the son didn't hear his mother. He was listening to his playlist and then realized he hadn't taken the dog out for a walk.

>> Maybe he thought that the dog needed a walk and that he would be back in time to take out the trash.

When we are behaviorally specific, we can see because it is observable to all, that the boy's mother is downstairs, she shouts up the stairs for the son to take the trash out, the boy walks the dog, and his father takes out the trash. That is being behaviorally specific. We would need to interview the boy as to whether he had heard his mother, and if he had, why had chosen to walk the dog instead? Some may say, "Well why are you so gullible, clearly the boy was trying to get out of his chore." DBT says not so fast. Unless this is a pattern of behavior where we do know the intentions and motivations of others, in the absence of all other information, we should assume the best in others. Use Worksheet 3–3 to practice being behaviorally specific.

Worksheet 3-3   Being Behaviorally Specific

PRACTICE

Consider words that are used to describe your behavior, or ones that you use to describe other people's behavior. Are they behaviorally specific? In other words, would someone who is watching the interaction see the same thing? What is the impact when you assume intention?

In the absence of any other information, have people called you manipulative, gamey, attention-seeking, lazy, or other behaviorally non-specific words? Or have you called others uncaring, abandoning, cheating, lying, and so on? Consider this as you answer the following questions.

1. Words used about my behavior.

    What the specific word was.

    _____

    _____

    What my observable behavior was.

    _____

    _____

    The impact on me because of the word used.

    _____

    _____

(continued)

Worksheet 3-3 *(continued)*

The impact on me when the other person misconstrued my intention.

_____

_____

2. Words I use about others' behavior.

What is the word I use?

_____

_____

What I actually know and see about the situation.

_____

_____

_____

The impact of my making incorrect assumptions based on my interpretation.

_____

_____

The impact on the relationship.

_____

_____

Does Every Problem Need a Solution?

The short answer is no. Now that you have established ways to identify problems and ways to think about solutions, this book being about dialectics, you also need to consider if every problem you have actually needs a solution. Here are some questions to consider:

>> **Does my problem need a solution?** The purpose of this step is to be as clear as possible in articulating the problem. For instance, say that you feel excluded from a group of people that are not close friends, but their social media posts show that they always seem to have a lot of fun. You are very happy with your current group of friends, but you are envious of the others' lifestyles. You say, "The problem is that I don't get invited to go out with others." Ask yourself these questions: "What is my desired outcome? Do I want to be invited to go out with them? Do I want to leave my current group of friends? Do I want my friends to be more fun?"

>> **Is solving this problem consistent with my long-term goals?** What are your long-term goals? How do friendships factor into achieving them? Will solving the problem of being excluded from a group of people that you are not particularly close to get you closer to your dreams? Is there any way in which solving this problem could be helpful to you? Maybe by clarifying who your true friends are? Maybe realizing that what looks great on social media is not always that much fun? Finally, how will you go about implementing the solution to this problem?

>> **How important is this problem in the bigger scheme?** Ask yourself: "Of all the things going on in my life right now, is this the problem that I want to spend all my time trying to solve? Do I have the energy and resources to solve this problem?"

Perhaps it looks like fun that the other group is going out every night, but that's an expensive endeavor, and maybe you have classes or work early every morning, so you might not have the emotional and physical energy to be out all night. Another consideration is if there is any further downside to solving the problem. For instance, you have a great group of friends, but you are envious of the other group's lifestyle. Might you be compromising important relationships with the group you are close with in order to feel more connected with the other group?

>> **So, do I need to solve this problem?** Now, you can answer this question with a clearer head. Of course, you can self-validate that it's not fun to be left out of certain situations, and yes, you might find it problematic that you are excluded, but in the bigger scheme of your life, not every problem is one that needs to be solved.

Not all problems need to be solved. Use Worksheet 3-4 to consider whether the problems you're experiencing actually need to be solved.

REMEMBER

PRACTICE

Worksheet 3-4   My Problem Is. . . .

Do you need to solve a specific problem? When you are considering whether a problem is not essential to solve, go through the following steps.

1. Define the problem in terms of specifics.

    _____

    _____

    _____

2. Is solving this problem consistent with my long-term life goals? If no, why not? If yes, why so?

    _____

    _____

    _____

3. Of all the things I am facing right now, is this a critical focus, needing resolution in the bigger scheme of things?

    _____

    _____

    _____

4. Do I have the emotional, mental, and physical resources to solve the problem?

    _____

    _____

    _____

5. Will solving this problem make my life dramatically better?

_____

_____

_____

6. Are there any downsides to solving the problem?

_____

_____

_____

7. So, is this a problem I need to solve? Do I need to solve it right now?

_____

_____

_____

Identifying Your Goals

Everyone has goals. For some people, these are very clear and established early in childhood. Others, however, take time to evolve. Whether it's the little girl who wants to be a doctor, the little boy who wants to be a plumber, or another child who is not sure, but as they reach adolescence, know what they *don't* want to do, and instead that they are interested in helping people, even if they don't know the specifics. Then there are people who do mainstream type jobs, such as working in a bank, a post-office, a hospital, a gardening shop, and so on. Others want to do jobs that are not as mainstream: teach parachute jumping, work on llama farms, fix old typewriters, and so on. The bottom line is that everyone has some goal.

REMEMBER

As it pertains to DBT, it is important for you, and, if you have a therapist, for them to know what your goals are because there is a second element to identifying goals and that is to identify your psychological goals. If there are psychological problems that are getting in the way of your overall life goals, clarifying your mental health goals is key.

Marsha Linehan applied dialectics to goal setting. She shared the following schema, which she called the *Goal/No Goal dialectic*:

> What motivates us is having our own individual goal. However, in the moment, in order to attain that goal, we focus not on the goal but on the steps necessary to attain it.

Say your goal is to reach the top of a mountain. You start hiking. If all you do is keep your eyes on the summit, you will likely have a dangerous outcome if you stray off the path, miss a rock, trip over a tree root, and so on. You may also lose motivation and focus when the mountain top continues to seem so far away. Since you have a goal, it's better to now let go of it and instead focus on each little step. Figure 3-1 illustrates this dialectic.

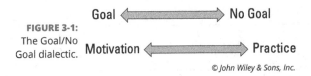

FIGURE 3-1:
The Goal/No Goal dialectic.

© John Wiley & Sons, Inc.

So having a goal motivates you, but you let go of the goal and do the little things to attain it. Rather than being mindful of your long-term goal, you are mindful of each step along the way.

WARNING

However, there is an important caveat to this approach. Sometimes, a person's mental health concerns are so overwhelming that setting longer-term goals seems impossible to even contemplate. In these cases, addressing their mental health issues should be the first goal. If you find that your mental health problems are impacting your life in such a way that you cannot set goals in any capacity, solving these mental health problems has to be your only goal. Use Worksheet 3-5 to work on your own lifegoals.

PRACTICE

Worksheet 3-5   My Lifegoals Are. . .

(If you don't have these goals yet, no need to worry. You can come back at a later point in time and fill these in.)

1. My short-term goals and what I need to do to achieve them.

   _____

   _____

   _____

2. My long-term goals and what I need to do to achieve them.

   _____

_____

_____

3. Are my mental health problems interfering with my goals? Y/N

_____

_____

_____

4. Do I have to address my mental health needs before pursuing my goals? Y/N

_____

_____

_____

5. Should my goal at this moment in time be to address my mental health problems?

_____

_____

_____

Short-term goals

The concepts of short- and long-term are relative. For some people, short-term means by tomorrow, and for others, it means in the next few years. There is no exact definition, so you have to determine what short-term means to you. Also, for many people, short-term goals are tied to long-term goals. For instance, one person might say, "My long-term goal is to be a social worker." Then that person might follow up with, "My short-term goal is to review social work programs."

However, for another person who is struggling with strong emotions, their long-term goal might be to apply to social work school, and their short-term goal might be to get out of bed and face the day effectively.

When it comes to mental health concerns, short-term goals can include going to therapy every week, attending group every week, completing all the DBT skills modules, using skills coaching, and completing all the assigned homework.

Long-term goals

Again, one person's short-term goals are another person's long-term goals. Generally speaking, however, long-term goals include life aspirations such as:

>> Buying a home in a community that is right for you

>> Developing a long-term relationship

>> Having a rewarding job

>> Contributing to a retirement plan for the long-term

>> Deciding on advancing your academic qualifications

When it comes to mental health, long-term goals can include a focus on overall health, such as:

>> Committing to regular exercise and balanced eating

>> Staying off mood-altering drugs

>> Getting regular physical checkups

>> Applying DBT skills to situations beyond ones that cause you stress as a way of staying generally effective

>> Establishing healthy, supportive relationships

Use Worksheet 3-6 to identify your short- and long-term goals.

PRACTICE

Worksheet 3-6   Clarifying My Short- and Long- Term Goals

Define what short-term and long-term mean to you and describe how can you expand on your short- and long-term goals.

1. Short-term for me is _____ (hours, days, weeks, months)

2. Long-term for me is _____ (days, weeks, months, years)

3. In reviewing Worksheet 3-5, my short- and long-term life and mental health goals are as follows.

Short-term life goals:

_____

_____

_____

Long-term life goals:

_____

_____

_____

Short-term mental health goals:

_____

_____

_____

Long-term mental health goals:

_____

_____

_____

REMEMBER

If your mental health problems are so debilitating that the idea of setting short-or long-term life goals seems like an impossibility, your mental health goals should be your priority.

Making a Commitment to Change

There are times when a parent brings their child to DBT, or a partner accompanies their loved one to a DBT session, and says something like: "They are living an unhealthy life, and they need to exercise more and smoke less." Now it would be wonderful if the child or partner agreed to this; however, just because someone else has a goal for you, does not mean that it is your goal, and certainly people are very rarely committed to change things that they don't want to change.

In some circumstances, the consequences of not changing are so significant that even if the person does not want to change for themselves, they will change for the health of a relationship. For instance, say a person says, "My loved one is drinking excessively. I saw my relatives die from alcohol related diseases, and the thought of this happening to my loved one is devastating. If they don't get help, I can't stay in the relationship; it is too painful for me."

It is possible that the partner really enjoys drinking and is not committed to changing this behavior, but the thought of losing their loved one may make them reconsider.

The key to success

The bottom line is that in order to change, it has to be your goal. Also, you can't just have the goal of change; you have to be committed to change and all that it entails, particularly when the going is tough. Think about the example of the person committed to climbing to the top of the mountain. It's not only on the relatively easy sections that they need to move, but during the difficult sections as well, if they want to attain their goal.

Research shows two important things when it comes to commitment:

>> **People who are committed to treatment and change do better than those who are not.** That applies to all aspects of medical treatment, exercise regimens, diets, and so on. It might make sense that this is true, but science verifies it as well.

>> **People don't have steady states of commitment to behavior change in the same way that they don't have steady states of energy or hunger.** Sometimes, people *are* committed to new behavior, but things get in the way, and they resort to older behavior.

If you live in a place that has snow, imagine that you are cross-country skiing. It is often easier to ski in the tracks of another skier than to make your own, especially when you are exhausted. Your mind will similarly find it easier to do old behaviors when you are tired. DBT recognizes that everything is in constant change, and this is true even of commitment. The DBT assumptions that "at any given time, a person is doing the best they can and yet need to do better, try harder, and be more motivated to change," accepts that a person might be committed while still needing to try harder. There is no linear path to recovery and the dialectical path fundamentally requires the dialectical movement between acceptance and change strategies.

REMEMBER

You can only commit to change things in your power. If you are committed to being more emotionally regulated, that is within your power. If you are committed to ending global warming, of course, you can do everything within your capacity and advocacy to do your piece, but you cannot commit for everyone else, as that is not in your power.

Worksheet 3-7 helps you reflect on the elements of your life that get in your way *and* that you can control.

Worksheet 3-7   I Am Fully Committed To. . .

PRACTICE

Reflect on the elements of your life that are getting in the way of attaining your goals, honoring your sense of self, setting personal limits, and so on. What, within your power, are you committing to change?

1. Commitments to change that are mine, independent of whether or not others support me.

_____

_____

_____

2. Conditional commitments: Commitments to change that I make that are not that important to me but are important to the important people in my life, so that overall, they are worth committing to.

_____

_____

_____

3. Behaviors or actions that I am not (currently) committed to change — ones that I feel would compromise who I am and what my values are.

_____

_____

_____

Barriers to commitment

So, if people want to change, why don't they? Many people who enter DBT have tried other types of therapies that weren't helpful. They feel that they talked about their problems for years, but nothing changed. One of the barriers could be therapy fatigue or skepticism that anything is going to work. Specific to DBT, however, many people worry that their level of suffering is so profound that four seemingly simple skills can't possibly change anything. Let's break this down a little more, because if there are barriers to committing to DBT, there are barriers to committing to the various skill sets. What are these barriers?

Barriers to mindfulness

In order to commit to DBT, you have to commit to the core skill of DBT, that being mindfulness. The reason is that all skills used mindfully, including mindfulness itself, are more effective. Some feel that mindful self-care is selfish, or even trivial in the context of all suffering. However, you have to start somewhere.

Another barrier is recognizing that mindfulness is needed but that you just don't have the time. You don't realize that the only time you have is now. Perhaps you are drinking a cup of tea, but here's the thing; you can drink your tea mindfully!

Others feel embarrassed or awkward by some of the mindfulness practices. "I am not going to sit in a lotus position and chant!" you might exclaim. Here's the thing. You don't need to! Sometimes sitting quietly and focusing on the breath allows for the intrusion of painful memories of a traumatic past. Not all mindfulness practices, at first, work for all people. There are infinite practices, and if one does not work, you can try another. Think of it like exercise. Just because others enjoy biking doesn't mean that you have to bike. You can jog, walk, do sit-ups, swim, and so on.

Another barrier: You simply don't know where to start — you don't have a teacher, and it just seems like too big a concept.

Barriers due to mental health conditions

Another set of barriers involves certain mental health conditions that hijack attention. For example, some people have attention deficit hyperactivity disorder (ADHD) or attention deficit disorder (ADD), which makes it difficult to pay attention. People who struggle with ADHD and ADD benefit from mindfulness practices. If you suffer from ADHD or ADD, you can break down your practice into a few minutes at a time while you increase your ability.

Barriers to interpersonal effectiveness

For many people who come to DBT, their experience of relationships has typically been complicated. Perhaps they experienced invalidation as a child. Or perhaps they have felt used in friendships or romantic relationships. Some people feel that they don't know what to ask for. Others feel that they do know what to ask for but don't know how to do it effectively. Others might feel that the only way to get their point across is to raise their voice. Some feel that they don't know how to say no, or that they say yes too readily. Many feel that if they don't acquiesce to the demands of others, they will end up feeling lonely and never have anyone in their lives.

Interpersonal effectiveness teaches you how to say no, how to be validated, how to set personal limits, and how to stick to your values. It can be scary to say no the first time, so it can be scary to even think about practicing relationship skills. For others, barriers include the experience that their words don't matter, that it is easier to simply shut up, that they don't deserve anything anyway, and other obstacles that tend to make people feel worse about themselves and actually lonelier in the long run. Finally, and like with all new life skills, the practice of anything new — including interpersonal effectiveness and relationship skills — takes energy, and you might feel that you are spent.

Barriers to emotion regulation

DBT was developed for people who have problems with emotion regulation. The idea that you could possibly control powerful emotions like rageful anger, unrelenting jealousy, and profound sadness can seem impossible. It can feel that because of the family you live with, you will never be able to control your emotions. Your family triggers a lot of your reactions. It might feel that the skills make sense for people with small emotions, but that yours are so big that no new behavior will ever control them. Unhealthy behaviors such as self-injury, drug use, or excessive spending often have such a powerful effect on reducing strong emotions that the idea of practicing skills that are not as powerful seems like a bad option. Some feel that strong emotions are what they know, how they get their points across, and that if they calm down, they won't know how to assert their needs effectively.

Barriers to distress tolerance

The ability to handle stressful situations without resorting to dangerous, maladaptive, or self-destructive behavior, is one of the clearest indicators of mental health. Life will be difficult for every person on earth at some point in time, and our task is to navigate these moments as effectively as we can. And when we cannot, to then tolerate the stress as effectively as we can.

For some people, the idea of practicing distress tolerance means giving up behaviors that have worked, even if temporarily, in the past. Riding the urge to act on an unhealthy behavior and instead tolerate the moment can seem nearly impossible. It can also feel exhausting to tolerate one difficult moment after the next, especially when difficult moments seem to come frequently. At times, the practices in the distress tolerance skills can seem trivial or even invalidating. "My girlfriend just broke up with me and you are asking me to breathe, listen to music, and do some gardening? Are you kidding me?"

REMEMBER Remember that you are coming to DBT therapy because whatever you have done up until now has either not worked or only temporarily worked, and you need longer-term solutions. In order to develop better solutions, you need to be able to tolerate difficult situations without making an already painful situation even more painful.

Worksheet 3-8 helps you reflect on your personal barriers to attending and practicing DBT therapy.

Worksheet 3-8   My Barriers to DBT Therapy

PRACTICE Think about the things that are getting in the way of you practicing any of these skills. Other than your worries about the DBT skills and format, is there anything else that is a barrier to your starting DBT?

1.   What are my barriers to engaging in DBT or any other type of therapy?

_____

_____

(continued)

_____

_____

_____

2. What are my barriers to the practice of mindfulness?

_____

_____

3. What are my barriers to the practice of interpersonal effectiveness?

_____

_____

4. What are my barriers to the practice of emotion regulation?

_____

_____

5. What are my barriers to the practice of distress tolerance?

_____

_____

_____

Overcoming barriers

DBT has some skills that therapists use in order to overcome the barriers to commitment, and although they are typically considered therapist strategies, that does not mean that you can't use them yourself. The following sections describe the main approaches to addressing ambivalence in commitment. You can do these on your own or with your therapist.

The use of pros and cons

Consider the pros and cons of DBT treatment. What are the pros and cons of not doing the treatment? Use the following grid. Now look at your long-term goals. What do your pros and cons tell you about what you should do?

Complete this pros and cons list and circle the items consistent with your long-term goals.

	Pros	Cons
Doing Treatment		
Not Doing Treatment		

Play devil's advocate

This is harder to do on your own, but ideally you gently argue against doing DBT treatment and ask yourself something like, "Am I sure I'm up for this treatment? It's a lot. Maybe I should wait for a month and then decide." Reflect on this idea and see what your gut tells you.

Foot in door, door in the face

This will almost always be done with a therapist. Rather than asking you for a lifetime of not engaging in self-destructive behavior, they ask for a smaller commitment, say a month or two weeks. For many people, a smaller commitment feels far more doable. Consider the mountain analogy used earlier in the chapter — the top of the mountain may seem too far, but a tree 200 yards up the path may seem more manageable.

With the door in the face approach, the therapist asks for more than the patient could likely do, and then, when the patient agrees to a more manageable request, closes the deal on the commitment to the more manageable task.

Connect the present to prior commitments

People are much more likely to trust that they can do something hard if they have done something hard before. Look back on your life and think about the hard things that you have done. Did you commit to complete a difficult academic course, sports camp, or language or music lessons? If you did, remind yourself that you can do hard things because you committed to and completed hard things in the past.

If, on the other hand, you had a difficult time completing your commitments, know that if this is the first commitment that you ever complete, it is likely to be one of the most rewarding ones you will ever do in your life. Use Worksheet 3-9 to contemplate past accomplishments.

PRACTICE

Worksheet 3-9   Past Accomplishments

Look back on your life and think about the hard things that you have done. Have you ever committed to something hard and completed it? If so, describe what it was. How did you do it? What got you through? Describe all the circumstances, people, and your own character traits that allowed you to do so.

_____

_____

_____

_____

Freedom to choose in the absence of alternatives

Imagine you are on holiday, your hotel hosts a great breakfast buffet, and you have all the choices you could possibly want. Now, imagine that the next morning, you wake up late and head down to the restaurant, and the choices left are foods that you barely like and many that you dislike. Or, on the third day, you wake up with barely a few minutes to go, and the only thing left is a kale smoothie, and you know that everyone tells you that kale is great for you, but you really dislike kale. It's obviously wonderful when there are plenty of choices in life, but at times, there are not that many, and sometimes only one. You have the freedom to choose, but sometimes, drinking the kale smoothie is better than going hungry. Worksheet 3-10 can help you identify your choices for therapy.

Worksheet 3-10   Making a Choice

PRACTICE

Is DBT or some form of therapy being recommended to you? Y/N

If so, is it your only choice? Y/N

If not, what are your other choices? What are the consequences of rejecting all your possible choices?

_____

_____

_____

_____

Generating Hope/Cheerleading

The problem that many people encounter with some forms of mental health treatment is that the outcomes are not always as clear. If someone needs to have their wisdom teeth taken out, you will know if they have been taken out within an hour. Or, if you have pneumonia, you will know within ten days if the antibiotic has worked. But for many psychiatric medications, for instance, it can take more than six weeks to know whether or not if they have worked, and another six weeks to know if a new one is helping. That is a long time to suffer if you are depressed.

DBT is great in that it has a lot of research behind it, and there is not so much guesswork. If you have difficulty regulating your emotions, DBT has emotion regulations skills. If you have difficulty in relationships, DBT has interpersonal effectiveness skills. If you have difficulty tolerating difficult moments, DBT has distress tolerance skills. If you struggle with being present and spend a lot of time worrying about the future or ruminating about the past, DBT has mindfulness skills.

So, here you go! This treatment really works for many of the struggles that have gotten you to DBT! And we know many others, who have struggled similarly and benefited tremendously from DBT! You got this!

IN THIS CHAPTER

» Moving beyond your first reaction

» Regulating your breathing

» Sensing your space

» Setting limits

» Reacting with intention

Chapter **4**

Being Intentional

Y ou now know a lot about the big picture of DBT. The following chapters take you deeper into the practice of DBT. This chapter focuses on understanding the reactions that show up when you have unwanted and painful thoughts or strong emotions. Sometimes the reactions can feel so automatic that you don't feel that you have a choice; however, there are ways to change how you react, especially if the way you react has led to negative consequences.

Moving Beyond Your First Reaction

Reactions don't come from nowhere. For many people who come to DBT, their behavioral reaction to emotions, or impulsivity, is what ends up being problematic. Reactions are critical to human survival. Without reactions, we wouldn't know to run away when something is threatening us. That is exactly what happened to the species of bird known as the dodo on the Island of Mauritius. In the late 1500s when the island was discovered, the sailors landing on the island were hungry, and they found a species of flightless bird, one that looked like a meaty pigeon, and it provided a great meal. Historical reports show that the dodos living there had no fear of humans, as they had never seen humans before, and the dodos were herded onto boats and used as fresh meat for sailors. In fewer than 100 years, a species that had survived for 8 million years went extinct.

Reactions are important to our survival! When we are — or feel — threatened, we tend to react. When threatened, most people experience the emotion of fear together with the thought that something bad or dangerous is going to happen, and the fear then drives anxiety or worry.

Anxiety and worry are more than just concepts, they are the body's biological and physical response to the threat and the fear. When a person feels threatened, it sets off a chain of events that starts with the release of stress hormones from the brain into the blood. Those hormones are messengers that go to different parts of the body — such as the muscles, the gut, the heart, and the lungs — in order to bring about specific physical changes to prepare the body to take action.

REMEMBER

Almost anyone who has taken introductory psychology knows of the so-called "flight, fight, or freeze response." These responses allow someone, hopefully, to deal with the threat. You run away, you fight back, or you freeze in place without moving so that you are not detected.

Reactions are what the body does, and they can feel automatic. However, you do have control over them. You actually have a lot more control than you think, but you have to learn to slow down.

Taking a breath

When people feel threatened, typically, their heart and breathing rates increase. The body is setting off alarms that something is wrong. This happens whether there is something actually wrong or not. An analogy is a fire drill alarm versus an actual fire alarm. The alarm sounds exactly the same whether there is an actual fire or not. Being able to distinguish between the two is critical. If there were a fire, you wouldn't then walk back into your house. During a drill, you would complete the drill and then walk back into your house because you know there is no fire.

Just because your body is sending you alarm signals does not necessarily mean that there is something wrong, but nevertheless you have to pay attention. Ideally, you should slow down and review the facts of the situation — one powerful way to do this is to slow your breath.

REMEMBER

While a fast heart rate and quick breathing are not necessarily dangerous, they can leave you feeling exhausted, and they may be telling you that there is danger when there isn't any actual danger. This means that you're more likely to react with intense anxiety, excess emotion, or even go into attack mode.

To move beyond your first reaction, you have to experience changing something you do every day, and practicing with your breath is a portable and ever-present way to notice and then change your reactions.

Regulating your breathing is like turning off the fire alarm. It involves slowing your breath rate and the manner in which you breathe. This section describes one way to do it, but there are many other methods for regulating your breath, and you can always practice the one that works best for you. You can do this anywhere — whether you are sitting on a chair, lying in bed, or even sitting at your office desk:

1. **Breathe in slowly through your nose (if possible) to the count of four or five.**

2. **Hold your breath to the count of two or three.**

3. **Slowly release your breath through pursed lips to the count of seven or eight.**

4. **Pause for a few seconds and then slowly repeat the cycle for two minutes.**

Once you slow and deepen your breath, you are, in effect, training your nervous system to be less reactive and anxious. Over time, you will notice that your overall stress level goes down.

Observing an urge

When people are experiencing intense and painful emotions, their desire to end the suffering is strong. With this desire can come the urge to act, and sometimes the actions are problematic — for instance, the urge to hook up with a stranger, the urge to self-injure, the urge to drink, the urge to misuse drugs, the urge to spend excess money, and so on. What acting on these urges has in common is that it (might) bring some immediate relief, but these behaviors are problematic and tend to exacerbate whatever pain you are feeling. In the end, acting on these urges doesn't solve anything because you aren't facing the painful emotions.

Here's the thing: the fact that you have an urge does not mean that you have to act on it, but it can feel nearly impossible not to. There is a powerful way to override the need to act on an urge, and it is known as *urge surfing*.

Before exploring the skill of urge surfing, there are a few things you need to know about urges:

>> Urges rarely last long, unless you continue to engage with them through the practice of focusing in on them, ruminating, giving them undue importance, or justifying them. *They will pass.*

>> Suppressing an urge by trying to distract yourself, denying it, or fighting it will make it stronger and more powerful.

>> Typically, as the urge to do something increases, it can feel as if it won't end until you give in to it.

>> The best way to get rid of such urges is to allow them to pass by observing them without acting or giving in to them.

Why surf an urge?

There is an interesting but not surprising characteristic of brain function: you get stronger at whatever you repeat and weaker at whatever you don't repeat. Ruminating on an urge makes the urge stronger. If you practice *urge surfing* (that is, observing urges without acting or giving in to them until they pass), your ability to urge surf without acting on the urge will get stronger.

By practicing urge surfing, you can learn to engage with urges in new ways. You learn that by riding them out, they will eventually subside.

Here is a way to think of urge surfing: Have you ever watched a surf competition on TV? You see the surfers on their surfboards on a relatively calm sea. Then a wave starts small, increases in size, and eventually breaks. The surfers who ride the waves know that the wave they are riding will eventually get smaller and reach the shore. Urges are like waves that you can surf. So how do you urge surf?

Learning to urge surf

TIP

The practice of urge surfing starts with mindful observation, and you can always use a mindful breathing practice such as the one explained earlier in this chapter.

Once you have settled into your breath, follow these steps:

1. **Notice your thoughts and label them as such.** Urges are thoughts. They are not actions. The urge to spend money is different from actually spending money. If you notice that your urge is intensifying, bring your focus back to your breath.

2. **Next, notice the way in which the urge impacts your body.** Notice any physical sensations associated with the urge. Do you feel any tightening in your muscles? Do you notice feeling warmer? Do you notice any unease or nausea? Is your breathing faster or more shallow?

3. **As you observe your urge, repeat the process of observing your body sensations.** Try to notice what happens to your body sensations as you observe your urge. Notice what happens to the body sensations if you try to fight the urge. Now notice what happens if you simply observe the urge without trying to fight. As you observe the urge, you might notice that it rises before it subsides and becomes more manageable.

4. **Once the urge becomes more manageable, repeat the cycle of observing it.** Each cycle of observing should take only a minute or so. Notice what happens to the urge through each cycle of observation. If it helps, visualize yourself riding on a wave with the wave being your urge.

TIP

Only surf one urge at a time. It is easier to carry one ten-pound weight than two ten-pound weights. Trying to do too much at a time can be exhausting and will make you less effective. The way to practice is to start noticing urges that don't cause you too much distress. For instance, you could do a body scan and see if you notice an itch. Observe the urge to scratch it, but don't. Or if you are sitting, observe the urge to shift positions in your chair, but don't.

5. **Tell yourself that rarely is anything so important that it has to be acted on immediately.** You can always wait an hour before acting on any urge. Give yourself some time.

6. **Now that you have resisted the urge, recognize your effort.** Once you have ridden out the urge, sit in the knowledge that you can do it again.

Sensing the space

In order to be intentional, you have to have to distinguish between what is you and what is not you. If you are an emotionally sensitive person, it may be difficult to distinguish between self and non-self, and that is because emotionally sensitive people tend to be emotionally porous and, sometimes, the emotions of others are the ones that you feel.

TIP

Another important thing to notice is whether you react to everyone's emotions or only to certain people. Some people have such heightened emotional sensitivity that they feel any emotion in the room. For others, their emotional porousness is limited to interactions with significant loved ones. It is key for you to notice and attend to the circumstances and the people who elicit significant emotional reactions.

WHAT DOES "SAFE" MEAN IN DBT?

In order to feel *safe*, you have to know what the red flags are for you and be able to set limits. One way to do this is to pay careful attention to the moments when a situation or person triggers anxiety or discomfort.

The word *safe* can mean different things to different people, and it can mean different things to you in different contexts. Putting on your seatbelt is a safe behavior. Removing matches so a child can't reach them makes the environment safer. In terms of psychological safety, this could be the freedom to express what you are feeling without the fear that you will be judged — or bullied or rejected.

It can also mean physical safety, where you feel that you are in a place in which you won't be physically attacked, assaulted, or touched in appropriately.

It can also mean all of the above. When you use the word *safe*, it's important to recognize what it means to you.

First, let's consider your personal and psychological space, the one that people regard as theirs. Think about your experience of having someone else in your physical or psychological space. Maybe your physical space has been violated and you have been physically hurt, even traumatized, or maybe you have been emotionally hurt.

One important aspect of space is to think about who is allowed in your space and who is not. There are all types of spaces and situations. There is your home space, friendship space, workplace space, school space, family space, intimate space, and so on, and distinguishing between these and who belongs in each space is key to an overall sense of safety. Use Worksheet 4-1 to identify the different spaces in your life (home, friendships, work, and so on), and then use Worksheet 4-2 to identify the different people in your life.

PRACTICE

Worksheet 4-1   My Spaces

What are all the different spaces in your life (home, friendships, work, and so on)? This worksheet is for you to detail these as clearly as possible, and then to notice in which of these spaces you feel safe, anxious, content, and so on.

1.   Space 1 and my emotions in that space:

_____

_____

_____

(continued)

_____

_____

2. Space 2 and my emotions in the space:

_____

_____

_____

_____

3. Space 3 and my emotions in the space:

_____

_____

_____

_____

4. Space 4 and my emotions in the space:

_____

_____

_____

_____

Worksheet 4-2   My People

Repeat this exercise by considering the various people in your life. Think about the people in your life and then think about how comfortable, anxious, happy, or afraid you are around them.

1.   Person 1 and the emotions I experience when I am with them:

_____

_____

_____

_____

2.   Person 2 and the emotions I experience when I am with them:

_____

_____

_____

_____

3.   Person 3 and the emotions I experience when I am with them:

_____

_____

_____

_____

(continued)

4. Person 4 and the emotions I experience when I am with them:

_____

_____

_____

_____

Letting go of attachment

Holding on to things that happened in the past or to that things in the future will go a certain way can cause you to suffer. It's healthier to accept that things might be different than what you want them to be and, despite this, you have the capacity to manage what comes. This approach can allow you to live a more effective life (see Chapter 9 for more about acceptance and non-acceptance).

REMEMBER

Much of suffering stems from *attachment*. Think about something from the past or a future aspiration that is causing you to suffer. Ask yourself what you are holding on to. Attachment comes in many different forms:

>> For instance, say that you are upset with someone because of their actions. You are attached to what you wish they had done or who you want them to be rather than fully accepting that they, as you, are who they are.

>> Say that you are ruminating on the comment a coworker made in the office. You play the comment over and over in your mind, and in so doing, you are bringing something that happened some time ago into the present moment. Why is it that there may have been many wonderful comments, but the harsh one is the one you are attached to?

>> Say that you wanted to run a marathon, but after a certain distance, you gave up. Of course, if you had been training for a long time, you would be disappointed. However, if you don't let this go, it is a manifestation of attachment to a different outcome.

We would all love for many things in the world to be different from how they are, but they are not. They are the way they are and what has happened to you is what has happened. Ask yourself if your attachment to things being a certain way is causing you to suffer. If you accept that not letting go is what causes you to suffer, then the answer must be to let go, right? Right! Just let go.

However, this is easier said than done. But this is true of any new idea or skill. Say you don't speak French. Someone tells you that in order to speak French, all you have to do is practice. Again, that is obvious, but the actual learning will take months and years of effort and practice.

Learning to let go is the same. It takes practice. Sometimes, when our minds are attached to something, we might not want to let go. Maybe you are attached to a romantic partner coming back to you. They left you months ago and are with someone else, but you hold on to the hope. Holding on to the hope does not change reality, and in fact, it makes it worse because each day of your partner not coming back is another day of suffering. You are attached to your partner not having left you, to them not being with someone else, to the hope that they will come back. You are attached to wanting things to go your way.

So, if the solution is to let go, how exactly do you do that? Start by working though Worksheet 4-3.

Worksheet 4-3 Targeting My Attachment

PRACTICE

How do you let go of attachment and clinging to past hurts and situations? Think about something from your past that is no longer happening right now that you are having a hard time letting go of. This worksheet helps you work through letting go. Be kind with yourself as you go through this exercise. Letting go of attachments rarely comes easily.

Accept this current moment for what it is: If you ruminate about the past, you are turning this moment into yesterday. But yesterday has gone. If all you do is spend time repeating what happened yesterday, you are effectively planning on making yesterday last forever. You are making yesterday permanent. Does this sound familiar?

1. Write about what you are attached to and how you are repeating the past by holding on to it.

    _____

    _____

    _____

    _____

2. Practice telling yourself that right now is enough. You have no idea what tomorrow will bring. It is possible that tomorrow will bring some painful circumstances like the loss of someone you love, the loss of a job, and so on. But the moment to deal with those things is then, not now, especially if in this moment, those things haven't happened. Right now is enough. Are you worrying about what might happen rather than what *is* happening?

    Write down what you are worried about and ask yourself if what you are worried about *is actually* happening or whether it is a worry thought.

    _____

    _____

(continued)

_____

_____

_____

3. Practice being fluid and flexible. Remember that you are constantly changing and grow-
   ing. You are not the same person you were a year ago, or a month ago, or even yesterday.
   You might feel the same, but you are not. Clinging to or attaching to something as if it
   will never change is like grasping an ice cube and imagining it will stay frozen forever.
   Change may feel slower and faster at times, but it is constantly happening. Practicing
   flexibility over rigidity will help. Ask yourself if you are holding on to the past as if it were
   a permanent thing happening right now.

4. Write the moment down and then practice being flexible with the thought by moving
   from what happened to right now, the present.

_____

_____

_____

_____

_____

_____

5. Throw yourself into the present moment. Sometimes when we suffer, we wallow in suffering, focusing all our attention on the source of our suffering. But there is also joy in the
   moment, even if it feels as if the only thing that matters is what is causing you to suffer.
   Does it help to focus on only that thing? Are there things that you can do right now that
   bring you some joy? This is not a cure, but it will lessen the intensity of the pain.

Consider whether all you are doing right now is focusing on the cause of your suffering. What are some things in the present moment that bring you some joy?

_____

_____

_____

_____

6. Don't be certain you know the outcome. Ask yourself how certain you are about the outcome of letting go. Are you sure you will be eternally miserable, that you will not be able to live happily, that you can't possibly let go of this attachment? How many times in your life have you done difficult things and you still survive. Remind yourself that you are stronger than you think. Of course, letting go will be painful and you can certainly validate that, but don't cling to the idea that you won't be able to manage.

Write down all the certainties you have as to what will happen when you let go of this attachment.

_____

_____

_____

_____

7. Remind yourself that you can't change the past. No matter how much you rethink the past, no matter how much you punish yourself for it, no matter how much you refuse to accept it, the past will not change. You are the only one who can torment yourself, and you are the only one who can give you the peace that you need.

Write down the ways in which you are trying to change the past.

_____

_____

(continued)

_____

_____

_____

8. Actively examine your attachment. If you are clinging to a past hurt or attached to a specific outcome, for example, holding on to a grudge or resentment, imagining getting into your dream school or getting your dream job, ask yourself why you are holding on so tightly. Of course, you can have aspirations. But if you turn these things into something that if they don't happen you will be devastated, ask yourself what the attachment is about.

    Write down some of the things that you are strongly attached to and ask yourself why you are so attached and what would happen if you weren't as attached.

    _____

    _____

    _____

    _____

    _____

9. Recognize that you can't know the future with certainty. Every day is filled with uncertainties. You can decide that you want to do something tomorrow but then something interferes with that plan. The restaurant is not open, your friend is not available, you catch a head cold, your sister wants to see you. Focusing solely and obsessing about the plans for tomorrow wastes your present moment because you are inserting all the hopes and worries about a moment that is not here in this moment. There are no guarantees as to how anything will play out, but you can choose to be present today and make the best of this moment. This does not mean that you shouldn't make plans. You need to recognize that there is no certainty that the plans will turn out as you expect them to and who knows, they may turn out better than you expected.

Write down a plan that you are fretting about and all the things that you are worried might happen. Identify the parts of the plan that you have very little control over.

_____

_____

_____

_____

_____

_____

10. Name your emotions. Strong and painful emotions can feel unbearable; however, avoiding the suffering only leads to more suffering. In Chapter 7, you learn how the skill of SUN WAVE can help you name your emotions. Feel the emotion, validate it, observe it, and express it. Doing so will allow painful emotions to pass more quickly than when you try to cling to them or avoid them, hoping that they will go away. Even if you want to stay angry or sad, limit this to a certain amount of time, especially when holding on to your anger, envy, jealousy, or sadness is causing you pain.

Write down any strong emotion you are feeling and consider whether you are hanging on to it excessively.

_____

_____

_____

_____

_____

Letting go of toxic relationships

The practices in the previous section may be helpful for letting go of objects and experiences, but what about letting go of an attachment to people who don't enhance your life?

REMEMBER

Very few people on the planet are all good, or all bad, and even the people who have not been the ones you needed in your life have some redeeming qualities. Some of the kindest people in your life have things that they struggle with. Move away from all-or-nothing.

How do you let go of attachment and clinging to people who aren't healthy for you? The ones who are not there when you need them, who only show up when you are doing well, who are solely focused on themselves, or who have said and done (and continue to say and do) hurtful things? Worksheet 4-4 can help.

WARNING

Before you end a relationship, make sure that this is a wise-minded decision. (Chapter 6 talks in great detail about the wise mind.) If you tend to be impulsive in your break-ups, you might end your relationship in the midst of emotional dysregulation. Determine what works in the relationship and what does not. If, upon reflection, the issue is minor, even if it caused you significant distress in the moment, breaking up might not be the right thing to do.

PRACTICE

Worksheet 4-4   Targeting Toxic Relationships

This worksheet is similar in format to the previous worksheet, where you work on letting go of attachments. Be kind with yourself as you go through this exercise. Letting go of people who you have been very connected to can be extremely painful.

1. You can be a friend to yourself. Sometimes the reason we attach to others is because they enhance our sense of self-worth. You have redeeming qualities. Think about the things that you like to do, and treat yourself to them as if you are treating a friend to those things.

    Write down the things in your life that bring you joy and treat yourself to those things as if you were a friend. (For instance a meal, a walk, a book, music, and so on.)

    _____

    _____

    _____

    _____

2. Remember that you are *not* the other half. You've heard people say, "this is my 'better half'" when discussing relationships. You are not the half of anything. You are a whole and possibly have many relationships. You are not a fraction. You can hold someone close to your heart without thinking that you would be nothing without them.

Write down the people in your life where you turn yourself into a fraction of who you are.

_____

_____

_____

_____

_____

_____

3. There is more than one other person in the world. Ask yourself if you have limited your-self to only one or two friendships. Have you turned one person into the entire world? You may feel unseen and unknown but there are many other potential connections in your life. Stay open to the possibility of connecting with others.

Write down whether you have limited yourself to just one or two people and then identify a few others (at your work, school, place of worship, and so on) that you can imagine connecting with.

_____

_____

_____

_____

_____

4. Ask yourself what you are afraid of. Often, people hold on to relationships because they are afraid of what will happen if they let go. Will they never find any connection? Will they be alone forever? Will they only be able to find hurtful people?

(continued)

Worksheet 4-4 *(continued)*

Write down what you are afraid of by letting go of this relationship.

_____

_____

_____

_____

_____

_____

5. Practice opposite action to love. In Chapter 7, you learn about the skill of opposite to emotion action. When it comes to love, you don't have to think of its opposite, hate, but instead, think about the many ways in which the person you love is flawed. You might be idealizing a person who has hurt you, and you want to counteract this idealization by reminding yourself about all the ways in which they have been unkind, unhelpful, and uncaring.

Write down all the ways in which this person has let you down or been hurtful. If you are noticing the urge to make excuses for hurtful behavior, notice those urges. The person may have many redeeming qualities; however, for the sake of this specific exercise, focus only on the hurtful and unwanted behaviors.

_____

_____

_____

_____

Reacting with Intention

Many people who come to DBT recognize that they are impulsive and that this impulsivity causes them problems in many situations. *Impulsivity* is the tendency to act without thinking about the consequences of your actions. Many times, if you look back on what you did in your wise mind, you know that your action had a high likelihood of being unhelpful or maladaptive. It can feel as if you have no choice — however, there is almost always a choice.

Considering different perspectives

When you are feeling desperate, you might only see things in a certain way and feel that you need to act on the specific urges that the moment is bringing you. However, is acting on your urge the only way? Can you see the situation from a different perspective? One immediate action you can take is to use the STOP skill in Chapter 9. Once you have done this, you can focus on the practice of perspective taking.

Perspective taking is the ability to look beyond your initial point of view. One way to think about it is to consider the specific situation you are in from an alternative viewpoint. To do this success- fully, you have to slow down enough in order to understand your thoughts, feelings, and inten- tions, and this is where the STOP skill can be a useful initial first step. Once you have stopped, there is a four-step approach to consider a different perspective, outlined in Worksheet 4-5.

EXAMPLE

For example, say you meet a new friend and invite them to dinner. They seem excited, yet they are shy, leaving all the plans up to you. You take them to your favorite steak house, and they seem very quiet and it appears they don't want to be there. You might interpret this as that they don't like you, but there may be many different interpretations of your new friend's behavior. Maybe they are vegetarian, and there are no veggie options on the menu. Maybe they have a significant headache but did not want to say anything because they were looking forward to having dinner with you. Maybe you took them to the same restaurant where they had a big fight with their brother and it brought back bad memories. The point is that if you only look at a situation through your perspective, you may be missing out on a different point of view.

PRACTICE

Worksheet 4-5   Targeting My Point of View

How do you take a different perspective on a situation so that you don't end up doing something impulsive and potentially damaging or inconsistent with your life goals? These steps are likely to be more successful if you have used the STOP skill (covered in Chapter 9) first.

1. Write down the situation and your thoughts, feelings, motivations, and intentions related to the situation.

_____

_____

(continued)

_____

_____

_____

2. Write down how your immediate action will achieve your short-term goals and your long-term goals.

_____

_____

_____

_____

_____

3. Write down if there are any other ways to see this situation. Are you acting on your own thoughts and urges? Do you understand all the facts of the situation? What other information do you need before you act on your urges?

_____

_____

_____

_____

4. Based on the results, rather than acting on your urge, write down alternative actions, or inaction, to address the way you are feeling.

_____

_____

_____

_____

_____

_____

Breaking free from rigid choices

There are many times when situations force you to make one choice or another. If you zoom out, your ability to accurately perceive situations is critical to your functioning. For instance, your ability to recognize whether your boss is happy or upset may be a key factor in deciding whether now is the right time to talk to them about a pay raise. A police officer interpreting whether you ran a stop sign with intention or by mistake might determine whether they give you a fine or not.

Sometimes, this binary way of thinking is directed inward. For instance, your present moment emotion may determine whether you will act on an urge or not. For many people who come to DBT, one of the common experiences is acting on mood. We call this *mood-dependent behavior*. Most people have to go to work whether they are happy, sad, or angry. For many people who come to DBT, strong emotions often determine whether they will do something or not.

We tend to think in binary ways, but the brain does not actually function that way. It only feels as if it does. In fact, there are gradations of feelings. You are not only happy or only sad. There is often more than just one feeling, and at a facial level, your face will express gradations of emotions. Think about it. When someone is happy, they might smile, or chuckle, or laugh. It's not only one single facial expression, but a range of facial expressions that manifest an emotion.

All-or-nothing thinking falls into a category of thinking known as *cognitive distortions*. Cognitive distortions are faulty thought patterns that typically end up with a person experiencing enhanced negative emotions and negative conclusions. If all-or-nothing is causing you to suffer, how do you stop thinking in all-or-nothing, black-or-white ways? (Chapter 11 covers much more about dialectics.)

One of the best ways to know if you are stuck in all-or-nothing thinking is by determining how certain you are about your conclusions and by recognizing that this certainty is based less on the actual data and information and more on simply how you feel. One of the best clues to this type of thinking is the use of words like always, never, fair, unfair, should, and shouldn't.

One of the biggest consequences of all-or-nothing thinking is that it tends to polarize complex situations, experiences, and people into simple categories, like good and bad or dangerous and safe. It is rare that anything is simply one quality. The fire that cooks your food is also the fire that burns your house down. The blade that someone uses to cut you might be the blade that a surgeon uses to operate.

Worksheet 4-6 can help you identify your own all-or-nothing thinking.

Worksheet 4-6   Tackling All-or-Nothing Thinking

Think about a situation where you were trapped in all-or-nothing thinking, one where you didn't have all the information, which caused you to suffer. Often there is a quality of certainty to this type of thinking. Review these practices and see if you can apply them to your life.

1. Relabel your thoughts. When you notice that you've assigned a single judgment to a person or situation, a judgment such as good or bad, take a moment to step back and label the judgment as a black-or-white judgment. If this type of thinking is automatic, the act of labeling the judgment pulls you out of this automatic thought process and activates the rational part of your brain. This is not permission to judge yourself for being judgmental. The task is to observe and label. You've now labeled the thoughts differently from "this situation/person is bad" to "I am thinking in all-or-nothing ways."

   Write down that situation that you are experiencing in black-or-white ways and then try to relabel the thinking about it.

   _____

   _____

   _____

   _____

   _____

2. Check the facts. Now that you have labeled what you are thinking, ask yourself if the way you are thinking is helpful or unhelpful. Ask yourself what evidence you have for your conclusion. What proof do you have? What are the facts of the situation? (It is absolutely

possible that your conclusion is, in fact, correct, and if it is, you want to make sure that it is based on facts and not simply on feelings.)

Write down the situation or identify the person that you are seeing in all-or-nothing ways and write down the observable facts that support your conclusion. You may want to ask a family member or friend for help. During this step, make sure that you are not using feelings as facts.

_____

_____

_____

_____

_____

3. Identify alternative explanations. For example, if you are certain that someone does not like you because they promised to call you and they didn't, identify alternative explanations other than that they don't like you. Did they forget? Did they have their phone with them? Are they sick? Did they get caught up at work? Are they worried about their pet, and so on? Write down the explanation that you came up with and write down alternative ones.

_____

_____

_____

_____

_____

Move from either/or to both/and

Many aspects of contemporary living demand that we define ourselves in one way or another. Are you a Yankees fan or a Red Sox fan? Republican or Democrat? Pro-life or pro-choice? Pro Second Amendment or against it? In DBT, there is a practice known as *Walking the Middle Path*, and it is the practice of recognizing that there is wisdom in all perspectives and that people come to their truth based on their circumstances, genetics, biology, experiences, and so on. Walking the Middle Path is embracing dialectics rather than succumbing to polarized thinking.

REMEMBER

Dialectics, one of the foundational principles of DBT, is about finding the synthesis between two seemingly opposite perspectives — recognizing the kernel of truth in other ideas while rejecting all-or-nothing thinking. Worksheet 4-7 can help you embrace the synthesis between two seemingly opposite perspectives.

PRACTICE

Worksheet 4-7   Embracing Both/And

Think about a situation where you were trapped in all-or-nothing thinking, and one where you simply could not see the other point of view or imagine how anyone could think differently from you. For example, someone could be intelligent AND spend no time studying. Or they could be kind AND hurtful when they get upset. Or a family member may be a good listener AND be too busy during the work week. The point is not to discount some quality about a person simply because another quality shows up. Write down the situation and consider these practices.

1. Embrace both/and. You can readily accept your position. Can you embrace the opposite position? You have to first accept that there is a problem with your perspective before you can change it. Acceptance is the dialectical opposite of change. You are accepting that you have a problem AND that it has to change.

    Write down a problem you have in the present moment and then use AND to recognize the opposite of that problem.

    _____

    _____

    _____

2. Examine the dialectics of who you are. Which parts of yourself seem at odds with each other? For instance, you might feel that you are unlovable AND yet feel desperate to be connected to others. You might feel that therapy feels impossible AND yet show up and try hard in each appointment. Write down some of the seeming contradictions of who you are.

    _____

    _____

    _____

Choose instead of react

We come full circle, and now is the time to integrate all of the skills you have learned in this chapter into the idea that you have choice in any moment. If you are behaviorally specific, you would see, because it is observable to all, that in this moment, you can choose rather than react.

Although it does not always feel as if you have choice, the truth is that your brain generates an urge. There is time between an urge to do something and the doing of that thing, even if it doesn't feel as if there is. Of course, if you have minutes or hours, you have the time to choose your action, but once you see that there is any time, you can expand the time by slowing down. In that space between the urge and the action is our power to make a decision, whether it is to act on the urge, not to act, delay the response, or choose a completely different response.

Earlier in this chapter, you learned about the skill of urge surfing. So, once you have stopped yourself from acting on an urge, how do you then choose what to do? You make choices based on your values, as Worksheet 4-8 shows.

Worksheet 4-8   Practicing Value-Driven Choices

You have used the STOP skill and surfed the urge to act. You have stopped acting on your urge! Congrats! How do you now make a choice?

1. Identify the decision. You need to make a new decision. Figure out what you wanted to solve by acting on your urge. This is the critical first step. Write down what you wanted to solve. Perhaps you wanted to avoid an argument with someone or avoid feeling pain related to the fact that your supervisor has switched your work hours. You avoid conflict at all cost, and yet your switch in hours means that you won't be able to attend a family gathering that you were really looking forward to.

    _____

    _____

2. Get the data you need to make the decision. Have you been acting on emotions? What information do you need to make the most helpful decisions, one based on facts? What information have you left out? Some of this information will come from outside sources. Rely on your emotions to the extent that they are helpful in making the decision, but do not rely solely on your emotions. What other information do you need?

    _____

    _____

(continued)

_____

_____

3. Remind yourself of your long-term goals. Is the decision your urge was telling you to make consistent with your long-term life goals and aspirations? What is your long-term goal and what are your values?

_____

_____

_____

_____

4. What are the alternatives to your urge? Once you have followed these, write down all the possible alternatives. Focus on alternatives that are consistent with your values and long-term goals.

_____

_____

_____

5. Evaluate each of the possibilities. Once you have reduced your list of possibilities to the ones that are consistent with your values and long-term goals, you need to evaluate them. How practical is each choice? How much support do you have to execute your plan? Write them down and list how practical each decision is. Prioritize the options in terms of feasibility.

_____

_____

_____

_____

_____

_____

6. Take action. Now that you have decided what to do, execute your plan. Write down the steps necessary to execute this plan.

_____

_____

_____

_____

_____

Chapter **5**

The Principles of Behavior

In this chapter, you begin to learn what makes you and the people around you continue certain behaviors and what makes you stop doing them. As we dive into the principles of behavior, you will see that — whether your behavior is adaptive or maladaptive, effective or ineffective — the same things determine if you will continue to do it or not. Understanding how this works can help you generate compassion for why you and other people do things that may get in your way or even hurt you, and it will also give you the key to unlock change and start new behaviors.

Taking the First Step

Marsha Linehan, the creator of DBT, did not create the behavioral principles. Rather, these principles are at the foundation of all behavioral treatments like DBT. You might have learned about these principles in high school or college psychology when you learned about Pavlov, his dog, and the bell experiment. For most people it takes a while to really grab onto these concepts, so you will likely want to review this chapter a few times. At first glance, this concept may seem easy. Slow down and really try to think about each principle and how it may be playing out in your life. Once you understand these principles, you will see them playing out everywhere. The key is not only understanding these principles, but staying curious and compassionate. Until you recognize these principles, they operate outside of your awareness, which makes changing behavior pretty hard.

You will find many definitions in this chapter. Take time to think about what each one means so that you can apply them to your life. Exercises throughout this chapter will help you understand the concepts and think about how they operate in your life right now. When you find yourself confused or frustrated by certain behaviors you keep doing or things that family members, loved ones, colleagues, and friends are doing, look back at these exercises and see if you can apply them to the behaviors you are seeing.

Understanding the Function of Behaviors

It may not always be clear, but behavior always has a function. It is your job to be curious and nonjudgmental as you investigate what that function or purpose may be. A good thing to remember is that if you feel absolutely certain about the function of a problematic behavior, you may be missing something, so keep that idea as one possibility and try to generate a few more.

For example, you (or someone in your life) may like school or your job and be motivated to do well and at the same time some days you may refuse to go or call out of work. On the surface, this makes no sense. If you like going and want to graduate or be promoted, why would you do the very thing that gets in the way of that goal? It is easy to assume that you are lazy or just don't care, but these judgments and assumptions shut off your curiosity and are typically wrong. Staying curious and generating hypotheses helps you more deeply think about the problem in front of you. Chapter 12 looks more closely at this situation and covers mood-dependent behaviors.

So why would you not want to go to work or school?

>> Perhaps you struggle with extreme anxiety and, while you set a goal to get up in the morning, you don't have the skills to manage your emotions and rely on avoidance to get through, so you stay in bed, losing sight of your long-term goals.

>> Perhaps you got into a disagreement with someone the day before and don't know how to navigate the situation.

>> Perhaps you had nightmares and only got a few hours of sleep.

>> Perhaps you have to advocate for something or say no to a request, and you don't know how. You might feel like the only solution is to avoid the conversation.

The first step to understanding behavior is to be curious and generate a few hypotheses (see Worksheet 5-1). Remember to stick to the facts when you are generating your hypothesis. Notice how we use the word "perhaps" to keep your mind open to possibilities.

Now that you have generated some hypotheses, think about whether any of them are helpful to you in determining what comes next (see Worksheet 5-2). Notice that when you generate nonjudgmental hypotheses, you have more information to generate the next steps. If you are thinking about someone else's behaviors, these hypotheses may just help you feel compassion and stay validated. This approach can help you avoid personalizing behaviors and avoid feeling hopeless.

Worksheet 5-1   Generating Hypotheses about the Function of Behavior

PRACTICE Practice generating hypotheses as to why you or someone in your life is behaving in a way that you don't understand or find problematic. Stick to the facts and keep your mind open to multiple possibilities. Try to understand some of your own problematic behaviors as well as others'. Do you notice any changes in how you feel after generating these hypotheses?

Behavior	Hypothesis #1	Hypothesis #2	Hypothesis #3
My best friend forgot to call on my birthday.	Perhaps since her mom is very sick, she had to take care of her and lost track of the date.	Perhaps she just isn't very good at remembering because she has forgotten a number of times and tends to forget our other friends' birthdays as well.	She doesn't enjoy celebrating her birthday and perhaps I haven't expressed how important it is to me for her to call and wish me a happy birthday.

Worksheet 5-2   Did These Hypotheses Generate Any New Emotions?

PRACTICE Write your reflections here.

_____

_____

_____

_____

_____

_____

Recognizing Reinforcers

Now that you have investigated possible functions of behavior, it is time to understand what makes them continue. Remember, this is a universal principle that affects all of us, even our pets! (Of course, using reinforcement with our pets can be a little easier.)

Reinforcers are consequences that follow a behavior (experiences including actions, feelings, thoughts, and even items) that result in an increase in a behavior in a particular situation.

Remember that the behavior can be adaptive or maladaptive, helpful, or unhelpful — if it is reinforced, the behavior will continue. There are two types of reinforcers — positive and negative. It is also critically important to remember that reinforcers are from the perspective of the person who receives them. What that means is that it must matter or have value to that person; otherwise, it is not a reinforcer.

Positive and negative reinforcement

This is one of the most important and most confusing concepts in the principles of behavior, or what is also called *behaviorism*. Part of the confusion with positive and negative reinforcement is that most people misuse these terms in everyday language, and they think positive means good and negative means bad. It is crucial to relearn these concepts. Draw on your early math skills and think not good and bad, but addition (+) and subtraction (-).

>> *Positive reinforcement* is when a behavior continues because something meaningful to the person is *added*. We call that thing a positive reinforcer.

   Positive reinforcers are the addition of something of value to the person that causes a behavior to continue. For example, if a manager gives a bonus for finishing a project more quickly, the bonus is a positive reinforcer. If a person thinks that the bonus is not large enough or they do not care about earning more money, it is unlikely that a bonus will increase the speed in which they complete a project and thus it will not act as the positive reinforcer. This concept is familiar to most people when training dogs and using treats as a positive reinforcer for new behaviors.

>> *Negative reinforcement* is when behavior continues because something is removed or *subtracted*. We call that thing the negative reinforcer.

   Negative reinforcers are the subtraction or removal of something aversive to the person that causes the behavior to continue. What is so powerful about negative reinforcers is that they give you relief! Most of the behaviors that bring people to DBT are at least partially reinforced using negative reinforcement. Again, this is not because these are "bad" behaviors but because they provide a sense of relief to the person. Relief has a very powerful impact on whether we continue or change our behaviors.

Negative reinforcers often provide short-term relief and are very powerful when it comes to our behaviors. When I have a headache, I take Advil and it makes my headache go away. Over time, I have experienced Advil seems to work more quickly than other pain relievers and as a result, I am more likely to take Advil in the future. Advil is the negative reinforcer because it provides quick relief and removes my headache. Use Worksheet 5-3 to investigate some reinforcers in your life.

Behaviors such as self-injury can be powerfully negatively reinforced. While it is a problematic behavior, most people say that when they feel emotionally overwhelmed, self-injury provides a profound sense of relief. This quick and powerful way to find relief is what can keep someone stuck in engaging in the behavior. That is, until they learn other skills to manage their emotions.

Although we are teaching these concepts discretely, there are often multiple reinforcers. These behaviors can have multiple positive or negative reinforcers and thus can be both positively and negatively reinforced at the same time. It is important to look for as many reinforcers as you can. For example, some people self-injure and get emotional relief (negative reinforcement) *and* find that the wound or the scar provides tangible validation of their suffering that they are not able to validate or express on their own (positive reinforcement) *and* find that it helps them connect with other peers in their friend group that self-injure as well (positive reinforcement). In this situation, there are at least three very important reinforcers that elucidate this behavior.

Worksheet 5-3   Positive and Negative Reinforcers

Now it is time to investigate some reinforcers in your life. Take a moment to think about a few of your own behaviors or behaviors that someone in your life engages in that you want to better understand. See if you can apply the principles of reinforcement to those behaviors.

Behavior	Reinforcer	Positive	Negative
Not doing laundry because I am depressed	Mom does laundry because she says it smells	Laundry done Not stressed Fewer self-judgments	Not stressed Fewer self-judgments

Extinction

At this point people, often ask how all this understanding helps us change behaviors? This is an excellent question and brings us to our next behavioral principle, extinction.

Extinction is the decrease and eventual elimination of a behavior by the removal of the reinforcers. Extinction is the most effective way to get rid of a problematic behavior in an enduring way; however, you must understand reinforcement, understand the most robust reinforcers, and then remove them.

Think about how extinction works using the laundry example provided on Worksheet 5-3. We know that when people feel depressed it can be very difficult to get things done because low mood, low motivation, and low energy really get in the way of taking care of yourself. One of the most helpful interventions is what we call *behavioral activation*. In DBT, we use the skill called *opposite action*, which we cover in Chapter 7.

Let's review what we understand from the worksheet example: Depression leads to not doing laundry, which results in no clean clothes, an aversive smell, stress about not getting it done, and self-judgments about all of it. The behavior of not doing the laundry is reinforced because eventually mom does the laundry, which provides relief from the task being undone, the smell is removed, and the teen gets a brief reprise from the self-judgments. Now that you are experts in reinforcers, you may have noticed that mom's behavior is also being reinforced because she does not like the smell of the laundry, so washing it provides her relief (negative reinforcement), and she feels like she is helping (positive reinforcement). Principles of reinforcement work in both directions!

Now we can put the behavior on extinction. In these types of situations, the mom's actions are often done with wonderfully good intentions; however, they prevent opportunities for opposite action and behavioral activation, which are healing, and they can perpetuate self-judgments. For some it can even lead to resentment, which can be problematic for the relationship. The depressed person might also feel increased shame from not doing laundry, which could fuel depression. Even though there are these problematic consequences of mom doing the laundry, the reinforcement — likely in both people — is more powerful, especially in the short term.

When you use extinction, when possible, you want to let the person know that you will be changing your behavior (removing the reinforcer). In this case, the mom should explain why she is no longer going to do the teen's laundry and why she has decided to change her behavior. Remember that stopping doing laundry is removing the reinforcer. If mom can tolerate not doing the laundry, eventually, the teen will complete it on their own. Extinction is challenging because reinforcement often comes outside of our awareness, and we get used to patterns and develop habits.

During the first stage of extinction, you will likely get no change in behavior or even an exacerbation of the behavior. For example, the laundry may go undone for even longer and smell worse. If the mom waits long enough, the teen will complete the laundry and likely feel a sense of mastery.

Remember, if the mom returns to the old behavior of completing the laundry, thereby putting back the reinforcer, she will very powerfully reinforce that if they simply wait their teen out, eventually they will do their laundry and be back to the beginning. This happens.

Having support during the process of extinction can be very helpful. Behavior takes time to change. You have to repeat this process over time and change will happen slowly and steadily. At times, you may see a return to the old behavior. Just ensure that you don't also return to the old behavior of applying the reinforcer and the new behavior will return. Reinforcement is the most effective way to create enduring behavioral change. Use Worksheet 5-4 to describe the behaviors you want to extinguish.

Worksheet 5-4   Extinction Plan

PRACTICE Describe the behavior you want to extinguish.

_____

_____

_____

Positive reinforcers:

_____

_____

_____

Negative reinforcers:

_____

_____

_____

Which reinforcers can be removed?

_____

_____

_____

What is my plan to remove them?

_____

_____

_____

(continued)

Worksheet 5-4 *(continued)*

Is this a situation with another person? I need to let them know.

_____

_____

_____

What is my plan to let them know (explain how will this benefit them — a positive reinforcer)?

_____

_____

_____

What support do I need to be able to stick with the plan?

_____

_____

_____

What will I do if I stray from the plan?

_____

_____

_____

Why is this plan a good idea?

_____

_____

_____

Understanding Shaping

Changing behaviors takes time. Sometimes you must reinforce approximations of the new behavior because the new behavior may be very hard to achieve. The concept of reinforcing smaller steps toward a new behavior is called *shaping*.

This very important concept lets the person know that while they have not achieved the desired new behavior, you do recognize that they are getting closer. This type of reinforcement encourages people to continue trying to achieve the new behavior. When you are using shaping, you want to remember that when you reinforce the smaller steps toward the behavior, you do not provide the *identified reinforcer*, but a smaller type of reinforcer such as some type of recognition, appreciation of their effort, or some smaller version of the identified reinforcer. Remember, any reinforcer you apply must be meaningful to the other person.

EXAMPLE

The *identified reinforcer* is the thing the person is working for, and *approximations* of the reinforcer are things that motivate the person to continue working to change the behavior but are not the final desired reward. For example, a teen may be working toward a later curfew if they can come in on time. The later curfew is the identified reinforcer. An *approximation* when they get close but don't get there on time may be recognition from the parent that they are working hard and provides motivation to keep trying to get home on time so they can earn a later curfew.

Many of our behaviors have been shaped and shaping even helps us develop some good habits. Teachers use shaping when they are teaching their students new skills. A parent of an anxious child can use shaping to help them attend school. At first, the child may only be able to attend for a few hours, even if the goal is to attend school for the entire day. Using *shaping*, the parents can provide some positive reinforcement at home, such as doing a special activity at home on days that the child is able to attend school. The child will get this reinforcer on days they attend and not get it on days they do not. At school, there may be time with a special teacher or increased time doing a desired activity on days they get to school.

Parents and teachers can continue to use shaping by providing additional reinforcers when the student attends a certain number of days in a row or a certain number of days per week. While the goal is to attend every day, shaping allows the child to get reinforced for steps toward the goal of attending school full time in a way that helps them remain motivated to practice their skills and ultimately get to school full time.

TIP

Many of you may use reinforcement to help complete tasks that are less desirable. This concept is called *self-reinforcement,* and you may be using it and not even realize. When you do this, you are controlling your own behavior in a way that provides motivation to do something or overcome something challenging. There are two ways people typically do this:

>> The first is using positive reinforcement to reward themselves for doing a task.

>> The second is using negative reinforcement, most commonly by reminding themselves about the relief that will come when the task is completed.

We used self-reinforcement frequently when writing this book! We would write and give ourselves positive reinforcers like going for a walk or getting a coffee or tea when we completed a chapter. We also used negative reinforcement, because meeting deadlines is important to both of us, and we both felt tremendous relief when we completed our chapters and got them in on time. Using self-reinforcement is a powerful tool for your toolkit.

Use Worksheet 5-5 to describe the behaviors you want to shape.

Worksheet 5-5   Shaping Behaviors

What is the behavior you want to shape? Why did you choose that behavior?

_____

_____

_____

What are some possible reinforcers?

_____

_____

_____

What approximations of the behaviors can you expect?

_____

_____

_____

What types of smaller reinforcers could you use?

_____

_____

_____

Pivoting on Punishment

Most people are much more familiar with punishment than with reinforcement. *Punishment* is when an undesired outcome follows a behavior that makes the behavior decrease or disappear. While there is a place for punishment, it is important to understand that it is much less effective in changing behavior in an enduring way than using reinforcement.

One of the dangers of using punishment too often is that the problematic behaviors tend to go underground, and the person learns ways to avoid the punishment by hiding the behavior or finding other ways to avoid the consequences. When you use punishment, it is important to know the difference between effective and ineffective punishment.

Effective punishment

Using effective punishment can, at times, be helpful. Many times, effective punishment comes from natural consequences. Natural consequences are expected consequences instead of ones you impose. For example, if you want to get a good grade but don't study for a test and get a low grade, the natural consequence is a low grade.

When you are imposing a punishment, it is helpful to remember some key things to ensure your use of punishment is effective:

>> **The punishment must be specific.** Don't be vague; clearly articulate what the problematic behavior was and what the punishment will be.

>> **The punishment must fit the crime.** This ensures that some learning can occur. For many parents it is easy to move directly to taking away things like phones, technology, or even access to a car, but unless that is in some way directly linked to the problematic behavior, it will not be effective.

>> **The punishment must be time limited.** Do not lay down a punishment that is so long that the learning gets lost. The younger the person, the shorter the duration of the punishment.

>> **The punishment must be livable to you.** Be sure that you are in a balanced state of mind or a wise mind when giving a punishment (see Chapter 6). Otherwise, you are at high risk of delivering a punishment that you cannot stick to or one that makes your life more difficult. Making your life more difficult has the consequence of you also feeling punished.

Examples of potentially effective punishments include these:

>> When a child does not complete their chores for the week, the parent adds an additional chore the following week.

>> Getting a fine for a speeding ticket.

>> A teacher giving a student extra homework for a week when they failed to complete their homework during a period of time.

Many people come to DBT with maladaptive behaviors that are powerfully reinforced. Natural consequences are some of the most powerful ways to change behavior. Sometimes that most powerful consequences arise and people experience these consequences as punishments due to their maladaptive behavior.

For example, some people who struggle with anxiety and constantly ask for reassurance end up losing friends because their friends find the frequent reassurance-seeking annoying. They might feel that their anxious friend does not express enough interest or concern in others because they are so focused on their own suffering.

Some people have shared with us that they have not gotten jobs or been able to be in performances due to their reliance on self-injury to cope. Other people have shared that because they struggle with their emotions and don't share things with their friends, they never feel close or connected to the people in their lives. These types of powerful natural consequences can feel quite punishing, and because they are so directly related to a behavior, sometimes they help a person contemplate change.

Ineffective punishment

When you fall into using ineffective punishment, everyone suffers. This type of punishment does not meet the criteria described in the last section and does not lead to behavioral change. It often leads to feelings of resentment or hopelessness, and it can send a message that you do not follow through with your consequences. Empty threats or punishments that are excessive and meaningless are ineffective and even harmful. Ineffective punishment does not leave the person with an understanding of what they did wrong or how to do something differently next time.

Examples of potentially ineffective punishments include these:

>> Suspensions from school

>> Grounding for an extended period of time

>> Taking everything away

>> Shaming

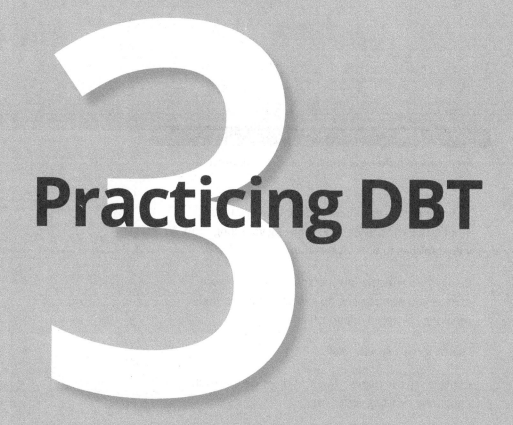

Practicing DBT

IN THIS PART . . .

Practicing mindfulness and focusing on the present moment

Trying emotion regulation by dealing with intense emotions in the present and reducing your long-term vulnerabilities to difficult emotions

Being more effective interpersonally, getting more of what you want, saying no and setting limits, and repairing disrupted relationships

Learning crisis survival skills

Considering the points of view of other people while equally recognizing your own

Thinking and behaving dialectically

IN THIS CHAPTER

» Understanding the benefits of mindfulness

» Considering your states of mind

» Working with your thoughts

» Setting up your practice

Chapter **6**

Mindfulness

M indfulness is the core skill of DBT and one of the four main skills modules. What makes mindfulness a core skill is that it is used in each of the other three modules. Dr. Marsha Linehan, the psychologist who developed DBT, found that adding mindfulness to her behavioral treatment was the most effective way to both alleviate suffering and help emotionally sensitive people change behaviors. The idea of starting to practice mindfulness can be overwhelming and confusing for some people. If this is or has been your experience, you are not alone. The good news is that DBT breaks down mindfulness into a skill that anyone can learn. Like all new skills, you must practice it to get better at being mindful.

In DBT, we find it helpful to think about mindfulness as a practice in attention. If you have strong emotions, this can be challenging, and you will see that learning to be mindful of your emotions and your thoughts is the first step in learning how to feel your feelings and choose effective skills to practice. Mindfulness will also help you be less reactive and less judgmental.

In this chapter, you learn and practice different ways to be mindful and pay attention as well as set up your mindfulness practice. Simply reading this chapter and completing these worksheets will not be enough to become more mindful. Mindfulness is like a muscle that you must exercise through practice. The more you practice, the more mindful you will become. Think about this practice as exercising your mindfulness muscle. The more you practice, the stronger the muscle gets. By the same token, when you stop practicing, the muscle atrophies. Remember, like all DBT skills, you need to practice mindfulness when you don't need it so when you are having a hard time and need to be mindful, you will have some muscle memory to help you be skillful!

What Is Mindfulness and What Are Its Benefits?

Mindfulness is a practice in paying attention and staying present, all without judgment. We know that the greatest hijacker of our attention are strong emotions. Strong emotions lead you to change your goals, say things you don't mean, make decisions you regret later, and keep you up at night as you worry about what is to come or regret what has happened. Most people live relatively mindless and habitual lives, but when you do that, you frequently miss out on many experiences and information. If you are an emotionally sensitive person, this can often lead to suffering. If you don't practice mindfulness, you may have never realized this! Paying attention will open your eyes to many things that you may have never realized.

There are many benefits to mindfulness:

>> **Helps you be more focused:** Mindfulness allows you to deliberately focus your attention; to notice when your mind has drifted to focusing on something that is not helpful or causing you suffering and give you the power to redirect or turn your mind to pay attention to something else.

>> **Calms your emotions:** Mindfulness helps you become less emotionally reactive. The more you practice mindfulness, the more you will be able to notice when your emotions are rising, observe them, and watch them decrease in intensity. The model of an emotion looks like a wave. If you can observe your emotion, it will rise in intensity like a wave, crest, and then slowly decrease in intensity like a wave meeting the shore.

>> **Gives you a feeling of choice over your behaviors:** When we teach mindfulness, we often tell people that mindfulness allows them to sit in the space between the urge to do something and do it. This is why mindfulness allows you to be less reactive. You will be able to observe an urge and make a choice instead of feeling compelled to do something. Before practicing mindfulness, many people feel like they just engage in behaviors as if there is little choice. When you pay attention, you can often find that point where choice is possible. This is very empowering!

>> **Improves your ability to relax:** The more you practice mindfulness, the more able you will be to shift your mind and body into relaxation. Because you are more able to focus your mind and are less reactive to your emotions, you can learn to ease yourself into a relaxed state more readily.

>> **Decreases your judgments:** We talk more about judgments later in the chapter. Judgments provide an overarching opinion about something, which is often oversimplified and leaves out important details. When you judge yourself and others in a negative way, it tends to create and perpetuate more painful feelings. People who come to DBT often struggle with negative self-judgments that fuel their suffering.

Understanding Your Own Mind

One of the most powerful things that mindfulness helps you do is pay attention and learn about your own mind. As you practice mindfulness, you will be able to step back and observe your thoughts, emotions, urges, motives, and memories. Mindfulness allows you to pause, observe, and make a choice instead of being dragged around by your thoughts and feelings and not even know that it is happening. Awareness is a powerful thing! You must also remember that our brains can do different things with the same information, and mindfulness helps you pay attention to what your mind does, as well as have fewer judgments about what other minds do.

WARNING Remember that your mind is a powerful source of information, and one of its functions is to produce thoughts and feelings. While you cannot control the thoughts and to some extent the emotions that your brain produces, you can control how you react and what you do with the information your brain provides you. Sometimes, the information is neither helpful nor accurate. Unless you learn to be mindful, you may live your life as if all this information is true, which can cause all sorts of problems!

DBT states of mind

So how do you pay attention to your mind? When you are emotionally sensitive and or have strong emotions, paying attention to your mind and emotions may be the last thing you want to do. At the same time, if you focus on your emotions, you will better understand yourself, your urges, and your behaviors.

One of the ways DBT helps you pay attention to your mind is by breaking the states of mind into three types:

>> Emotion mind

>> Rational mind

>> Wise mind

These states of mind are universal; we all have them. There are different situations during which being in a specific state of mind will help you be most effective. The goal is for you to be able to identify what state of mind you are in and move between the states, depending on what makes you most effective. Let's look more closely at each state of mind.

Emotion mind

Emotion mind can get a bad name because people who come to DBT often spend too much time here, but it is a very important state of mind. To best understand emotion mind, think about the metaphor of a pair of glasses. When you are in emotion mind, the lens of your glasses is how you feel in that very moment. In this state of mind, you engage with the world around you based on how you feel and not what you know. This is a fast-paced state of mind that is driven by the immediate, the right now. In this state of mind, you do not connect with what you know or things too far in the future.

You may have heard of *mood-dependent behaviors,* which is when you do things based on how you feel and when your mood changes, your behaviors follow. For example, when you are feeling good you can get to work, follow through on commitments with friends, and get things done around the house, but when your mood shifts and you feel more anxious, disappointed, or depressed, these things feel like they no longer matter or feel too hard to take on, and you don't do any of them. This state of mind can also lead to forgetting long-term goals for something more short term. If you spend too much time in emotion mind, it can lead to unintended or unanticipated consequences.

Many people ask what the point of the emotion mind is. The emotion mind is critical! There are times when having your emotions lead the way is important. If you are in danger, your emotion mind gives you quick information so you can act fast. If there is a fire or you are walking somewhere dark, you likely get that sense of danger that then makes you change your behavior quickly. Emotion mind can keep you safe or even save your life.

Emotion mind is also a wonderful place to be when you are falling in love or celebrating good news with someone you care about. It is also the state of mind to be in when you are grieving. The key with emotion mind is to know when it is effective to be there, when it is not, and how to shift to another state of mind if you need to. Catching your emotion mind before you move into action or make decisions can help you be more effective. See Worksheet 6-1.

Worksheet 6-1   My Emotion Mind Behaviors

Use this worksheet to list behaviors that signal that you are in emotion mind. In DBT, behaviors are not just actions but can also include your thoughts. Circle the behaviors that you can use as red flags to denote that your emotion mind is not effective at the time.

Emotion mind behaviors:

_____

_____

_____

Emotion mind thoughts or thinking:

_____

_____

_____

_____

Rational mind

The rational mind is the opposite of emotion mind. If you return to the metaphor of a pair of glasses, when you are in your rational mind, you see the world through the lens of what you know and *not* how you feel. While the emotion mind is faced-paced, the rational mind is a slow, logic-based state of mind. When you are in rational mind, you have access to all that you know to make slow, well-thought-out decisions. You want to be in rational mind when you are taking exams, working on things like your taxes or accounting, when you are solving logistical problems, or when you need to make decisions without your emotions involved.

WARNING

If you struggle with hard-to-manage emotions, you may feel like this state of mind is ideal, but remember that sometimes, making logical decisions without considering how you feel can cause problems as well. Sometimes, the emotional mind can be masked as the rational mind, and it can sound like a calm and clear logical argument, but when arguments are circular, or the other person cannot consider or be open to new information, the logic may be emotion minded. See Worksheet 6-2.

Worksheet 6-2   Times When I Need to Be in My Rational Mind

List situations when you realize it is important to be in your rational mind.

_____

_____

_____

_____

_____

Wise mind

The wise mind is the intersection of your emotion mind and your rational mind. When you are acting from your wise mind, you are considering how you feel and what you know. Like the rational mind, the wise mind is a slower paced state of mind. You must synthesize your feelings about the situation and the facts. These decisions are deliberate and rarely have unintended consequences. Many people feel like their wise mind is a place of all-knowing and deep-seated knowledge. These decisions are often difficult but will leave you with a sense that you made the "right" decision. Many people feel a deep sense of calm after a wise-minded decision, even if they feel sad or fearful of what is to come.

REMEMBER

Everyone has a wise mind. If you have not experienced wise mind, it is not that you don't have one, but that you may have trouble accessing it. Getting to know how you think and feel during all of the states of mind will help you develop mindfulness awareness of what state of mind you are in and how you can move from one state to the next.

Worksheet 6-3 helps you identify when you are in your wise mind, and Worksheet 6-4 helps build your awareness of your different states of mind.

Worksheet 6-3 How Do I Know When I Am in My Wise Mind?

Use this worksheet to identify your wise-minded thoughts and behaviors as well as how it feels in your body to be in your wise mind. Use these familiar signs to help develop awareness of your wise mind.

Wise-minded thoughts	
Wise-minded behaviors	
Wise-minded body sensations	

Worksheet 6-4 My States of Mind

Use this worksheet to fill in the Venn diagram with thoughts, feelings, behaviors, and body sensations that you can use to build your awareness of your different states of mind.

States of Mind

Reasonable Mind

Wise Mind

Emotional Mind

Mindfulness of current thoughts

As you become more aware, you will begin to pay attention to everything around you. It can be very helpful to learn to pay attention specifically to your thoughts because thoughts can be powerful forces that drive your emotions and behaviors. While paying attention to your thoughts can be challenging, it will also help you change your relationship with thoughts that are not helpful.

Being mindful of painful thoughts will help you practice radical acceptance (see Chapter 9). It is a wonderful thing to realize that you can recognize thoughts as thoughts, choose to believe them or not, and even choose to agree or disagree with them, all before acting on them. There is freedom in becoming aware of what you are thinking!

Here are the steps to practicing mindfulness of current thought:

1. **Notice the thought and label it as a thought.** Don't push it down or judge it, just watch it and let it pass through, like a cloud moving across the sky. Try not to get caught up in it. It can be helpful to say to yourself *I notice the thought that I am a failure,* or *I notice the thought that I can't do this.*

2. **Be curious.** Ask yourself questions like *I wonder where that thought came from?* Don't evaluate, just stay open. With practice, you will be able to laugh a little at some of your automatic ineffective thoughts. Don't grab on to thoughts and think about them, let them move on.

3. **Remember that you are not your thoughts.** Try not to move into action. Remind yourself that these are only thoughts. If they are painful, remind yourself that they will pass, and you have had different thoughts in the past. If your thoughts are from your emotion mind, remind yourself of this and that you also have wise-minded thoughts about whatever you are thinking about.

4. **Do not push down, block, or suppress your thoughts.** Stay open and let your thoughts move. Suppressing thoughts is one of the best ways to enhance the painful thoughts and emotions that come with them. Notice when you are blocking or avoiding thoughts, take a deep breath, and let them come. Embrace difficult thoughts or even be playful with them, maybe by saying them in silly voices or repeating them as fast as you can. Remember that they are just thoughts that you can watch and let go, even if they are painful!

Worksheet 6-5 helps you be mindful of your thoughts.

Worksheet 6-5   Mindfulness of Current Thought Practices

Use this worksheet to practice being mindful of your thoughts. Write down your observations.

1. Go to a park or a busy place and sit and watch the people around you. While you are watching, observe your thoughts. Each time a thought comes into your mind say, *I notice the thought.* . . . Write down some of the thoughts you notice.

   I notice the thought_____

   _____.

   I notice the thought_____

   _____.

   I notice the thought_____

   _____.

   I notice the thought_____

   _____.

   I notice the thought_____

   _____.

2. Think about something that happened in the recent past that made you upset. As you think about it, notice the thoughts that arise in your mind. Label them as thoughts and ask yourself these questions:

   Where do I think this thought came from?_____

   _____

   Why does it feel so important to me?_____

   _____

   Have I had this thought before?_____

   _____

   Can I let this thought go?_____

   _____

3. Consider a thought that comes up over and over again that you would like to be less consumed by. Now work with your thought by engaging with it differently, without invalidating your feelings.

   Say it really fast over and over in your mind. Record your observations:

   _____

   _____

   Say it really slowly like slow motion over and over again in your mind. Record your observations:

   _____

   _____

Working with your cognitive distortions

If you have any experience with Cognitive Behavioral Therapy (CBT), you are probably familiar with cognitive distortions or errors in thinking. While they are less formally a part of DBT, cognitive distortion comes with the emotion mind, so it is important to be familiar with it so you can keep on the look out, be mindful of these thoughts, and learn how to work with them.

REMEMBER

Because cognitive distortions are often driven by emotions in the moment, it is easy to believe they are true. Sometimes, the behaviors we do as a result can have negative consequences on our goals and relationships.

Here are some common cognitive distortions to be mindful of:

>> **All-or-nothing thinking:** This type of thinking is absolute; it is not nuanced — it is one thing or the other. This is a very *sticky* kind of thinking (in other words, it is easy to get stuck in this type of thinking and have a hard time challenging it or seeing any other perspectives or options). Example: *If I don't win the competition, then I have to quit my sport.*

>> **Jumping to conclusions:** When you jump to conclusions, you do not take into account all of the facts of the situation, and you draw a conclusion based on some of the information, often your own negative interpretations. Example: *I only got the promotion because they felt bad for me.*

>> **Overgeneralization:** This happens when you take one negative experience and generalize it into a never-ending pattern of loss, defeat, or negative outcomes. Keep a look out for words like always, never, everything, and nothing as a signal you may be falling into overgeneralization. Example: You answer a question in class wrong or make a suggestion at work that colleagues don't agree with, and you think, *no one values what I have to say; I am never speaking up again.*

>> **Disqualifying the positive:** You believe that the positive experiences don't count, so you reject them to maintain the negative. Example: If you receive a compliment from someone, you think, *they only said it to be nice; they don't really know me.*

>> **Catastrophizing:** This is very common when people are anxious. This is when you jump to the worst-case scenario or the worst possible outcome, despite how unlikely it is. Keep an eye out for "what if" lines of thinking as a red flag for catastrophizing. Example: *What if this relationship doesn't work out? What if I am alone forever and no one will love me?*

>> **Mind reading:** This is when you decide what someone is feeling (usually negatively toward you) without any evidence to support it. Example: *I feel like she hates me, so she must hate me.*

>> **Personalization:** This leads you to believe you are responsible for something that you are not and often leads to feelings of guilt or self-loathing. Example: *It is my fault that you didn't succeed.*

>> **Fortune telling:** You worry that things may turn out badly and you treat this worry or assumption as fact. Example: *I know that I won't ever find a relationship, so I am not going to date.*

>> **Emotional reasoning:** This leads you to believe that the way you feel is reality. If you feel it, it must be true. Example: *If I don't feel like a competent person then I will never be successful.*

Cognitive distortions are a tell-tale sign that you are operating from your emotion mind. As you become more mindful and skillful at mindfulness of current thoughts, you will be increasingly able to observe these cognitive distortions, label them, and either let them pass or challenge them. Worksheet 6-6 helps you identify your common cognitive distortions.

Worksheet 6-6   Working with My Cognitive Distortions

Use this worksheet to identify your common cognitive distortions, validate the emotion behind it, and then use your wise mind to challenge it.

Emotion Mind Cognitive Distortion	Validate the Emotion	Wise Mind Challenge
All-or-nothing thinking		
Jumping to conclusions		
Overgeneralization		
Disqualifying the positive		
Catastrophizing		
Mind reading		
Personalization		
Fortune telling		
Emotional reasoning		

Practicing Mindfulness

This section digs deeper into the nuts and bolts of mindfulness. Many people find the idea of mindfulness to be a bit overwhelming and hard to wrap their minds around. The two questions we get most often are:

>> What do I do to practice mindfulness?

>> How do I do it?

DBT answers these questions directly by teaching the *what* and the *how* skills of mindfulness. Once you understand and practice these skills, you will be on your way to becoming a mindfulness practitioner. The following sections review each of these skills and give you practices along the way.

The "what" skills

This set of skills answers the question: What do I do to practice mindfulness? Like many of the DBT skills, they are organized into the *what* skills, covered in the following sections.

Observe

The practice of observing is simply noticing using your senses. It is noticing all things — the environment around you, your body, your thoughts, and your emotions. When you observe, you just notice and do not react. You observe without words — your task is to simply be with the experience. It is not easy to simply observe, because we automatically label and judge things.

HOW TO SIT WHEN YOU PRACTICE

When you practice seated mindfulness, unless we tell you otherwise, find a quiet place and sit either cross-legged on the floor or in a chair with your feet on the floor. Turn off your cell phone or other distractions. Set your intention to practice mindfulness. Sit up straight so that you can breathe easily. Gently rest your hands in your lap, palms up or palms down. Try not to cross your arms or legs or hold tension in your body. Take a couple of deep breaths and bring your attention into whatever room you are in. Then take a couple breaths and turn your attention to your breath going in and out of your body. Remember, it is natural for your mind to wander away from the practice — your task is to catch it and gently bring your attention back. Now you are ready to practice!

PRACTICE

1. Notice an urge to swallow: Set up your seated practice described in the sidebar and spend a few minutes noticing the urge to swallow without swallowing. Notice the sensations and thoughts that arise.

    Observations:

    _____

    _____

    _____

2. Notice an itch: Set up your seated practice and spend a few minutes noticing itches without scratching. Notice the sensations and thoughts that arise.

    Observations:

    _____

    _____

    _____

3. Go outside and observe with your senses: Notice the air on your skin, the temperature, and the smells.

    Observations:

    _____

    _____

    _____

Describe

When you mindfully *describe*, you are putting a label to what you observe. You can do this with thoughts, feelings, sensations, or anything else you observe. When you describe, you only use facts. There are no opinions or editorials, just facts. You have used the describe skill when you are mindful of your current thought and you describe by saying, *I notice the thought that....* It can be very helpful to do this with emotions as well. When you label an emotion, you take the first steps in decreasing its intensity. You could describe your anxiety by saying, *I notice I am feeling anxious; my heart is beating quickly, and I am feeling hot.*

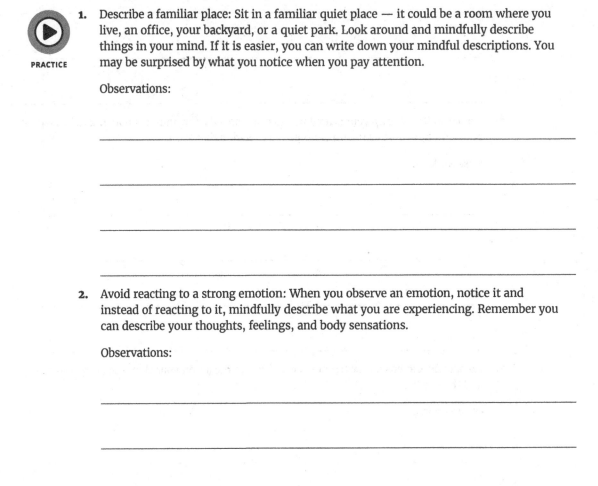

PRACTICE

1. Describe a familiar place: Sit in a familiar quiet place — it could be a room where you live, an office, your backyard, or a quiet park. Look around and mindfully describe things in your mind. If it is easier, you can write down your mindful descriptions. You may be surprised by what you notice when you pay attention.

   Observations:

   _____

   _____

   _____

   _____

2. Avoid reacting to a strong emotion: When you observe an emotion, notice it and instead of reacting to it, mindfully describe what you are experiencing. Remember you can describe your thoughts, feelings, and body sensations.

   Observations:

   _____

   _____

   _____

   _____

3. Describe a picture: Look at a photo, a magazine cover or ad, or photo in a newspaper and describe it mindfully. Remember, just stick to the facts.

Observations:

_____

_____

_____

Participate

This is a slightly different type of practice. When you practice participate mindfulness, you throw yourself fully into what you are doing and let go of self-consciousness. Self-consciousness and worry about what others are thinking prevents you from being present in the moment.

PRACTICE

1. Participate in a conversation at work, school, or with a friend: Set an intention to fully participate in a conversation. Notice worries or self-consciousness and commit to one-mindfully throwing yourself into the conversation.

Observations:

_____

_____

_____

2. Dance or sing: Find a place alone and try to fully participate in either dancing or singing. Notice any self-consciousness and see if you can throw yourself into the moment. Let go of how you look or sound.

Observations:

_____

_____

_____

3. Do an ordinary daily activity that you don't like: Pick an activity that you must do that you dislike, something like dishes, laundry, or a chore around the house. Now try to fully participate when doing it and don't get caught up in thoughts about not liking it, wanting it to be over, or why others are not doing this for you.

Observations:

_____

_____

_____

_____

The "how" skills

Now that you know *what* to do to practice mindfulness, you need to know *how* to do it. You will use each of the how skills when you are observing, describing, and participating. While the what skills are distinct practices, you will use each of the three how skills non-judgmentally, one-mindfully, and effectively when you are practicing mindfulness.

Non-judgmentally

Being non-judgmental is part of being mindful. If you can master this skill, you will notice many changes in your experience of yourself and others. Negative judgments about yourself and others can add to your suffering. It is not easy to let go of judgments. The world is very judgmental. So, what are judgments? They are shorthand descriptions. They allow us to take complicated concepts or experiences and pair them down into one word. We all use judgments! Examples of judgments are good, bad, ugly, pretty, stupid, creepy, awesome, weird, fair, unfair, and what should or should not be.

As you can see, judgments can be positive and negative. Judgments leave out information, and they also tend to shut down our curiosity. The goal is not to eliminate judgments completely, but to be very mindful of when to judge and when judgments are causing suffering.

You may be surprised at how challenging it is to be non-judgmental. Many times, your judgments are habitual and automatic. Mindful awareness of judgmental thoughts will help you learn when your judgments are effective and when they are not. Reducing your judgments takes practice. Remember — don't judge your judging!

PRACTICE

1. A magazine or newspaper photo: Find a photo in a magazine or newspaper and describe it non-judgmentally. Now describe it judgmentally. What do you see? Write down your mindful and non-mindful descriptions. What do you notice about each experience?

Descriptions:

_____

_____

_____

_____

Observations:

_____

_____

_____

2. A difficult emotion: Think about a difficult emotion and try to describe it when you are not experiencing it. Write down your mindful descriptions. Once you have practiced this several times, try this when you are experiencing the emotion.

Descriptions:

_____

_____

_____

_____

Observations:

_____

_____

_____

_____

3. A difficult situation: Think about a difficult situation you encountered recently. Now describe the situation non-judgmentally. Read your description. How do you feel about the situation now?

Descriptions:

_____

_____

_____

_____

Observations:

_____

_____

_____

_____

One-mindfully

Doing one thing in the moment is fundamental to your mindfulness practice. When you are one-mindful, you are doing one and only one thing at a time. This is the opposite of multitasking. Doing things one-mindfully has two elements:

>> Being fully present in the moment. Not getting stuck in the past or thinking about a future that has not happened.

>> Doing one thing at a time.

Most of us do a lot of multi-tasking and believe that it makes us more efficient. However, research shows that very few of us multi-task, instead we are rapidly shifting our attention, which over time tires our brain, makes us less efficient, and makes us more likely to make errors. This practice is one of full attention on only one thing in the moment.

PRACTICE

1. Choose an everyday task: Practice doing something you do every day, like washing the dishes, watching TV, or driving, and practice doing it one-mindfully. When your mind wonders, gently bring it back to the mindful task at hand. What do you notice when you do this activity one-mindfully?

   Observations:

   _____

   _____

   _____

   _____

2. Non-dominant side: Practice something you do with your dominant hand using your non-dominant hand. Think about tasks like brushing your teeth, putting your pants or shirt on, or writing the alphabet. What do you notice about your attention?

   Observations:

   _____

   _____

   _____

   _____

3. A conversation: Many people are not one-mindful when they talk on the phone or in person with others. Put your phone away, turn the TV or music off, and one-mindfully have a conversation with someone in your life. Does it feel different?

   Observations:

   _____

   _____

_____

_____

Effectively

This mindfulness skill is about doing what the situation needs — keeping your goals and the greater goals of the situation in mind and doing what works, even if it is different from what you want. One way to think about effectiveness is taking a step back and asking, *do I want to be right or effective?* We are asking you to turn your focus away from fair and unfair or who is right and who is wrong and look at what is effective and what works. Effectiveness can be very hard to practice when you are in emotion mind, which is when you need it the most.

Another way to look at mindfulness is the capacity to have focused attention, which we have talked about, and, at the same time, have expanded awareness. That is, you can be focused on something and at the same time remain aware of what is going on around you or the bigger picture.

TIP

To practice effectiveness, you first need to know what you want or what your goal is. Once you are aware of your goal and can articulate it, you need to step back and look for the most effective way to achieve it. You need to think about things such as:

>> Is the timing right?

>> Will this impact important relationships, your reputation, or how you think about yourself?

>> Is the goal achievable?

>> Will there be negative consequences?

>> Is it a priority over other things?

This has probably happened to everyone who drives. You are driving down the street, and someone looks like they are about to cut in front of you. If you don't slow down, they will hit you. While the other person's behavior is not right, the effective thing to do is to let them in instead of speeding up and trying to prevent them from cutting in front of you. Practicing effectiveness is not easy and requires you to practice awareness in making a decision that often elicits strong emotions.

Here is another example we hear a lot. We often hear from students that feel their professor owes them a point or two on an exam. Now, they absolutely are right about this point and deserve it; however, this is a difficult professor who tends to penalize students who confront them about their grading. This is a very difficult situation because the students deserve the points and should not be penalized for the professor's mistake in grading. In this situation, they are absolutely right. This student decides not to fight for the two points because they have an A in the class, and decide that maintaining the good relationship with their professor and getting all the participation points would be better for them in the long run. Practicing effectiveness can be very challenging; start with Worksheet 6-7.

Worksheet 6-7 Practicing Effectiveness

This worksheet asks you to practice effective is several areas of your life. Remember that practicing is the best way to get better at something, and that is no less true with mindfulness.

1. Effectiveness with food choices: Practicing effectiveness with food can be challenging. Practice making effective choices during the meal. This does not mean restricting, this means paying attention to food allergies or sensitivities, how much you eat, and what foods you eat. Be deliberate and mindful taking into account what food works for you, what makes sense given the occasion, and your long-term needs or goals.

Observations:

_____

_____

_____

_____

2. Effectiveness with goals: In the morning, review a goal for the day or the week. Make a list of how you will be effective that day in working toward your goal. Remember to make your plan considering whatever else you may have planned or need to do that day.

_____

_____

_____

Steps:

_____

_____

_____

Observations:

_____

_____

_____

(continued)

3. Effectiveness with sleep: Commit to acting effective around your sleep routine for three consecutive days during the week. How did you practice and what did you observe?

Day 1	Effective Behaviors	Observations
Day 2	**Effective Behaviors**	**Observations**
Day 3	**Effective Behaviors**	**Observations**

Setting a Routine and Building Your Practice

Incorporating anything new into your life means building a new habit, and the best way to do that is to set a routine so that you can practice the *what* and *how* skills every day. The first thing you need to think about is where and when you will practice.

While we are hoping that you will start to live your life more intentionally and mindfully, we would also like you to commit to a daily practice. Start at just five minutes and build from there!

TIP

It takes around ten weeks to build a habit. The best way to build a habit is to do the new behavior, in this case mindfulness, at around the same time of day and in the same place. Use Worksheet 6-8 to describe where you will commit to practice. Worksheet 6-9 helps you identify the things that get in the way of your practice and how you can address them.

Remember that building a new habit is hard. This is a great habit to have because it is one that will change your brain. Like all good DBT therapists, whenever we ask people to build new habits and change behaviors, we ask them to problem-solve any barriers they experience.

Worksheet 6-8   Where and When of My Mindfulness Practice

Using this worksheet to describe where you will commit to practice and what times of day. Be as detailed as possible and include any changes you may need to make to the space.

Where I will practice:

_____

When I will practice:

_____

Time of day:

_____

How long I will practice:

_____

_____

Worksheet 6-9   Problem-Solving Barriers to My Mindfulness Practice

Use this worksheet to identify the things that get in the way of your practice and how you can address them. These can be emotions, like fear, excuses, lack of time, or no place to do it.

Barrier	How Can I Address this Barrier So It Doesn't Get in the Way?
I don't have time to practice mindfulness.	I know I can find five minutes during my day when I wake up, during my lunch break, or before I go to bed.
It's hard to sit still.	I can start doing mindful breathing while walking.
I am afraid I am doing it wrong.	Mindfulness is a practice, and as long as I have something to focus my attention on and can catch my mind when it gets distracted, I have practiced mindfulness!

(continued)

Barrier	How Can I Address this Barrier So It Doesn't Get in the Way?

Chapter **7**

Emotion Regulation

E motion regulation is one of the four main modules of DBT. This chapter helps you learn to use your emotion regulation skills to identify and name your emotions, identify which emotions are primary and secondary, which are justified and unjustified, as well as understand the function of your emotions.

Practicing emotion regulation skills helps you decrease the intensity of your emotions as well as learn to reduce your emotional vulnerabilities. Learning to use your emotion regulation skills will help you begin to intentionally increase and decrease your emotions.

What Is Emotion Regulation and What Are the Benefits?

Many people who come to DBT are emotionally sensitive. As noted in Chapter 1, emotionally sensitive people feel things longer and deeper than the average person and tend to take longer to return to their emotional baseline when they are dysregulated. They also tend to have larger emotional responses to things they experience or are considered more reactive.

If you are a sensitive person, and you don't know how to regulate your intense emotions, you may often suffer. Many people who come to us for DBT ask if we can get rid of their emotions because they have caused them so much pain. We cannot rid you of your emotions (nor would that be good for you), but we can teach you skills to increase your awareness of your emotions and to intentionally modulate the intensity of what you feel.

If you are unable to consistently regulate your emotions, you are at high risk for your emotions taking hold and dictating your behaviors. These are *mood-dependent behaviors* (discussed in Chapter 12). When your mood is "good," you feel like you can go to work or school, see your friends, and get things done around your house, which are all important things to you. However, when your mood dips and you feel more challenging emotions like sadness, fear, anger, shame, guilt, disgust, or even jealousy and envy, suddenly the things that you want and need to do can feel less important or even impossible to get done.

As you practice the skills in this chapter, you will get hold of your emotions by increasing your awareness of them and more confidently applying skills to regulate how you feel. This way, your emotions will not interfere in your life but instead will help you live your life.

Understanding and Identifying Your Emotions

Learning to identify your emotions is the first step in changing the intensity of what you feel. This chapter builds on some of the mindfulness skills covered in Chapter 6 so you can better understand what you are feeling and what you want or need to do next. Being aware of your emotions can be challenging, but it provides clarity about what you can do to navigate your emotions more smoothly.

Finding the function of emotions

We said earlier that we cannot get rid of emotions, and we said that because emotions have three very important functions:

>> To communicate information to the person feeling the emotion

>> To communicate to and influence others

>> To motivate action

As you can see, your emotions are both critical and powerful! Emotions tell you about the world around you and how you feel about it. The first step in learning to regulate your emotions is learning how to observe them and name them. In fact, pausing and naming your emotions can begin to decrease their intensity. Sometimes, simply naming your emotion is the only thing you need to do to regulate it. Use Worksheet 7-1 to assess what you have learned from some recent emotions.

Primary and secondary emotions

You will experience many emotions throughout the day. Figuring out and labeling what they are may seem daunting. It is important to be able to distinguish your primary emotions from your secondary ones. As the name implies, primary emotions are the ones that you feel first, and secondary emotions follow.

Worksheet 7-1   What I Learned from My Emotions

PRACTICE

Take a moment and think about the last week. How did your emotions give you important information about the world around you, the people in your life, or the decisions you needed to make? Use this worksheet to log what you learned from your emotions over the last week.

Situation	Emotions I Felt/ Experienced	How the Emotion Served Me/What Function It Had
I overslept on a work day	Scared I would get fired Angry at myself	The fear made me get ready faster than I have before and helped me be only 15 minutes late. The anger at myself helped me realize that I need to work on my sleep and have a backup plan to make sure I wake up in time.

Primary emotions

You can think about primary emotions as the first emotion your brain produces based on information coming in from your five senses. Primary emotions last an average of 90 seconds. We like to think about these primary emotions similar to a neurological event — information comes in through your senses, your brain processes the internal or external experience, and produces an emotion to give you information. Primary emotions are hard wired and are associated with specific facial expressions that can be seen across cultures. Remember that one of the functions of emotions is to communicate information to yourself as well as to others.

There is much debate over the number of primary emotions. Some people believe there are four, five, eight, or ten primary emotions. Marsha Linehan, the creator and founder of DBT, referred to ten primary emotions — joy, love, sadness, anger, fear, guilt, shame, envy, jealousy, and disgust. The following sections look at each of these emotions in detail.

JOY

A feeling of pleasure, happiness, or contentment.

Joy prompts: Receiving good news or a wonderful surprise, accomplishing something, being accepted, being with people you like or love, doing things you enjoy.

Joy sensations: Urges to smile and laugh, feeling at peace, feeling energetic and excited.

Joy urges: Smiling, sharing with others, hugging people, jumping up and down, talking, and sharing.

LOVE

>> An intense feeling of deep affection.

Love prompts: Receiving something you want, need, or desire, feeling physically attracted to someone, sharing a special experience with someone.

Love sensations: Fast heartbeat, full of energy, warm, calm.

Love urges: Smiling, expressing positive feelings, hugging, holding someone, sexual activity, wanting the best for the person.

SADNESS

>> A feeling of sorrow or unhappiness.

Sadness prompts: Losing someone or something, death of a loved one, not getting what you worked for, being rejected, being excluded, hearing about negative events in the world, being isolated.

Sadness sensations: Low energy, heavy, hollow, empty, difficulty swallowing, dizzy.

Sadness urges: Hiding, crying, avoiding, acting helpless, withdrawing, giving up.

ANGER

>> A strong feeling of annoyance, displeasure, or hostility.

Anger prompts: Having an important goal blocked, you or someone you care about being hurt, having things not turn out as expected.

Anger sensations: Muscle tightening, clenching, feeling hot.

Anger urges: Wanting to hit, yell, throw, or hurt someone.

FEAR

>> A strong feeling that something or someone is dangerous or likely to cause harm or threat.

Fear prompts: Having your life or health threatened, flashbacks, being somewhere unfamiliar, having to perform in front of others.

Fear sensations: Fast heartbeat, lump in your throat, butterflies in your stomach, feeling clammy or nauseous.

Fear urges: To scream, to freeze, run away, avoid, cry.

GUILT

>> A feeling of having done wrong, failed an obligation, or crossed a personal value.

Guilt prompts: Doing or thinking something you believe is wrong or against your values, causing harm to someone or something you care about, being reminded of something you did wrong in the past.

Guilt sensations: Hot face, feeling jittery, hard to breathe.

Guilt urges: Avoiding, hiding, asking for forgiveness, trying to change the outcome.

SHAME

>> A painful feeling of humiliation or distress caused by the awareness of foolish behavior or behavior that crosses societal norms and leaves a person feeling ostracized or different.

Shame prompts: Being rejected by people you care about, having others learn you have done something wrong, being betrayed, being criticized in public.

Shame sensations: Pain in your stomach, sense of dread.

Shame urges: Avoiding, withdrawing, hiding, slumping.

ENVY

>> A feeling of discontentment due to the desire to have a possession, attribute, or quality that someone else has.

Envy prompts: Someone having something you really want, not feeling part of the in crowd, someone getting credit for your work.

Envy sensations: Muscles tightening, clenching, feeling hot.

Envy urges: An urge to get even, hating the other person and wanting them to fail, feeling motivated to improve yourself.

JEALOUSY

>> A feeling of uneasiness from suspicion or fear of rivalry, or fear of something deeply important being taken.

Jealousy prompts: A competitor paying attention to someone else, getting ignored by an important person who is talking to someone else instead, your partner flirting with someone else.

Jealousy sensations: Breathlessness, fast heartbeat, choking or sinking sensation, muscles tensing.

Jealousy urges: Threatening or violence toward someone else, asserting control, spying, clinging.

DISGUST

>> A feeling of revulsion or strong disapproval aroused by something unpleasant or offensive.

Disgust prompts: Seeing something dirty, observing or hearing of something that strips another person of their dignity, seeing something dead, observing or hearing someone acting with extreme hypocrisy.

Disgust sensations: Feeling nauseous, urge to vomit, feeling contaminated.

Disgust urges: To get rid of something, aversion to doing or being around something, to shower.

REMEMBER

Some of these emotions may be very familiar to you and others less so. Make sure to look closely at two pairs of emotions — guilt and shame and jealously and envy — as they are often confused and used incorrectly in common language.

Spend some time looking at this list. You can also refer to it when you are working on identifying your primary emotions. When you self-validate and validate others, you always want to search for the primary emotion.

Secondary emotions

Once you learn to identify your primary emotion, you will see how secondary emotions are the ones that get you stuck. In many ways, understanding your emotions would be easier if you didn't have to worry about secondary emotions. Secondary emotions are a result of thinking, judging, and invalidating your primary emotions. Unfortunately, it is your thinking about your emotions that causes emotions to last longer, feel more intense, and even add other painful emotions to an experience that was already painful in the first place. The problem with secondary emotions is that they can last for a long time — hours, days, months, and years. When you are stuck in secondary emotions, they have a way of self-perpetuating and leaving you more and more stuck. Misery is a great example of being stuck in a mix of secondary emotions.

EXAMPLE

Any primary emotion can also become a secondary emotion. For example, you are sad because you lost your job. You then begin thinking about all the other jobs and people in your life you have lost and may even start telling yourself you shouldn't be so sad. Your thoughts and beliefs about your sadness lead to more sadness. Here, you had primary sadness and now have secondary sadness.

What can be tricky is that your secondary emotions can be different from your primary emotion. Have you ever been cut off and the person nearly hit you when you were driving? Many people's first reaction is to get angry, but is that the primary emotion? No, most people feel fear when someone nearly hits their car when they are driving. It is not that anger does not make sense, it does, but it is not the entire story of the experience. Fear comes first and then anger happens very quickly for some people. When you pay attention and validate your fear, it will dissipate. When you focus on the anger (and the thoughts associated with it), you will find yourself fueling it, and it can last for hours or even days.

TIP

If you are experiencing an emotion for longer than 90 seconds (if it has not been prompted again), that is a good clue that you may be stuck in a secondary emotion. The more you practice identifying and labeling emotions, the more skilled you will be at focusing on the primary emotion and catching when you may be inadvertently doing things that get you stuck in secondary emotions.

Justified and unjustified emotions

Another thing to keep an eye out for is whether your emotion is justified or unjustified. This designation can feel judgmental, and it is not meant to be. All emotions are valid, but not all emotions are justified.

An emotion is *justified* when it fits the facts of the situation. The intensity matches the situation and how long you experience it fits the situation. People who are emotionally sensitive often feel things longer and deeper than the average person, so they are more at risk to have an unjustified emotion, which just means they are feeling it too deeply and for too long, which is getting in the way of how they want to live their life.

The skills in this chapter help you navigate unjustified emotions. When you notice an unjustified emotion, such as feeling scared in a situation that isn't actually threatening, it is very important not to invalidate or judge yourself. Strong emotions work this way, and it is a wonderful clue to use some skills. Later in this chapter, we introduce a skill that is particularly helpful in navigating valid but unjustified emotions.

Naming Your Emotions and Decreasing Emotional Suffering

Learning to identify your emotions is the first step in changing the intensity of what you feel. You build on some of your mindfulness skills that you learned in Chapter 6 to better understand what you are feeling and what you want or need to do next. Being aware of your emotions can be challenging, but it provides clarity about what you can do to navigate your emotions more smoothly. Consider why the following emotions are considered justified and unjustified:

>> **Justified anger:** I had a flat tire and was late to work.

>> **Unjustified anger:** I had a flat tire and was late to work and was so angry that I swore at the tow truck driver, was angry for the rest of the day, making it very difficult once I got back to work.

>> **Justified sadness:** My partner broke up with me, and I spent the weekend in bed, crying and focusing on self-soothing. I returned to work on Monday feeling sad and receiving support from my friends.

>> **Unjustified sadness:** My partner broke up with me and I stayed in bed all weekend, did not answer calls or texts, and could not go to work consistently the rest of the week due to crying and feeling so hopeless.

Reducing emotional vulnerability with ABC PLEASE

When you feel emotions intensely, it is important to learn ways you can make yourself less vulnerable and more resilient. When you come to DBT, it can feel like so many things are out of your control. One of the things that we love about the ABC PLEASE skill is that it is a place where you do have control.

We all have what we like to call an *emotional foundation*. Like the foundation of a house or building, it keeps the structure stable, especially when it is under stress. Your emotional foundation functions the same way. When your foundation is balanced, it is stable, and you are better able to manage and navigate the emotional hurricanes and tornados that come your way. For a sturdy foundation, you must be aware and practice your ABC PLEASE skill.

REMEMBER

This skill has two parts. The first part, ABC, includes more psychological things you can do to build a sturdy foundation. The second part, PLEASE, includes skills to regulate your physiology or take care of your body. To start, the following sections explain the ABC portion.

A: Accumulate positives

Dr. Marsha Linehan, who developed DBT, always said that we need to live an antidepressant life. That is, we need to actively seek out things that make us feel happy and joyful and not wait for them to just happen to us. We all need to have things in our lives that bring us joy, and it is our responsibility to take part in creating and paying attention to those experiences. When our mood is low and life gets stressful, these activities can be the first ones to go. Be mindful that — independent of your mood — you always need to keep working on bringing yourself joy. Your experiences of joy can be big and little. When you build positive experiences each day, you are building resiliency. We also know that when people are experiencing many painful emotions, they're more likely to miss or discount the more pleasant ones. By being on the lookout for positives, even small or fleeting ones (like someone letting you merge into traffic on a busy day), you are more likely to build a foundation that helps you weather difficult emotions.

B: Build mastery

Accomplishing things that are challenging has a positive impact on our mood. Each day we need to feel a sense of mastery by achieving something challenging and doing things we're good at. Some people can find this during school or work, projects around the house, hobbies, sports, learning a new skill, or working through a to-do list. Identifying long-term goals and creating a roadmap of small steps help people feel more competent, which solidifies their mood.

C: Cope ahead

Preparing for potentially challenging situations makes us less vulnerable to strong emotional reactions or ineffective behavior. To practice the *cope ahead* skill, follow these steps:

1. Mindfully and non-judgmentally describe the facts of the situation and the difficulty you might encounter. Make sure to stick to the facts before you move to the next step.

2. Decide what skill you will use if the situation arises. Make a chain of at least three skills as there are very few situations in which one skill will help you navigate a challenging situation ahead. Make sure you identify the emotion.

   You can use your SUN WAVE NO NOT skill, followed by some self-validation.

   If the emotions around the situation are very intense, you can look for some distress tolerance crisis survival skills (Chapter 9). Then, depending on your goal, choose a more change-oriented type of skill (emotion regulation or interpersonal effectiveness).

   If it is a difficult situation that you need to accept because you cannot change it, look toward the acceptance models (distress tolerance or mindfulness).

3. Visualize the situation you are planning for and how you will execute your plan. Repeat this step, paying attention to additional challenges that may arise or additional skills you may need to use. Rehearsal, even imagined, increases the likelihood that you'll follow through on the plan.

4. Think of the worst-case scenario. This is usually something you have been dreading, keeping you up at night, or avoiding thinking about all together. You may be stuck in a loop of "what-ifs." Take a moment to experience the feelings of your worst-case scenario coming true and then rehearse your plan and see if you need to adjust it to make sure it also addresses the worst-case scenario. The good news is that most of the time, the worst-case scenario does not happen.

The following sections look at the PLEASE portion of this skill.

P: Physical illness

Not feeling well physically impacts your mood and this seems particularly true for people who are emotionally sensitive. When possible, treat physical symptoms and be proactive. We are all more vulnerable when we are sick or are in pain.

Remember that this part of the acronym focuses on ways to work with your physiology or your body to maintain a strong emotional foundation.

REMEMBER

L: Lather, rise, repeat

While not part of the official PLEASE acronym, a group of patients we worked with at McLean Hospital decided to enhance the acronym by adding an "L," which we found very useful. They added the idea of *lather rise repeat*. They noted that when your mood is low it can be hard to shower and take care of your activities of daily living (ADLs). When you shower or bathe, it supports your mood, which decreases emotional vulnerability, especially when your mood is already low. While it was less popular, they also added *limit screen time*.

E: Balanced eating

Early in life, the link between eating and mood becomes very clear. You likely have heard the word or experienced the feeling of being *hangry*. When we are hungry or if our eating is out of balance (e.g., eating only "junk food"), we are often more irritable, judgmental, and impatient. Our emotions are more likely to hit us more intensely. Balanced eating includes frequency, amount, and the type of food. All of this impacts mood and increases emotional vulnerability when they are out of balance.

A: Avoid mood-altering substances

Not surprisingly, mood-altering substances by definition alter your mood. When you are practicing your PLEASE skills, pay attention to drug, alcohol, nicotine, caffeine, and even sugar intake. Remember, whether you use these substances responsibly or not, they all can have an impact on your emotional vulnerability. Sometimes the impact is within minutes and sometimes it lasts longer than a day.

S: Balanced sleep

You may be the most familiar with the impact of sleep on your mood. Healthy adults need on average eight hours of sleep each night and adolescents need between eight to ten hours. Going to bed too late, having nightmares, and frequently waking interrupts sleep and leaves you more vulnerable the next day. If you struggle with sleep, are just not getting enough, or are sleeping too much, you likely know that your experience of the world is very different compared to when it's balanced and consistent. For many people who come to DBT, balanced sleep is one of the hardest PLEASE skills to balance.

E: Exercise

You are probably familiar with some of the research on exercise and mood. The nice thing about exercise and mood is that most of us feel the positive impact during or right after we work out. The difficult thing is that when your mood is low, exercise can be one of the hardest things to do. The goal is to be able to exercise, independent of your mood.

WARNING

When working on your PLEASE skills, be mindful of the impact that one skill can have on another. PLEASE skills powerfully impact one another. If you are not careful and aware, when one falls out of balance, the others can follow like dominos. For example, when your sleep is out of balance, you feel too tired to exercise, so you drink an excess of caffeine and you don't want to cook, so you order food that is easy but doesn't support your mood. While the caffeine does help with energy, it makes you more anxious, and it's harder to fall asleep. Eek! The good news is that as quickly as your PLEASE skill foundation can crumble, you can rebuild it by simply getting one part of the skill back in balance. The others will follow, and you will feel an improvement in mood and a decrease in emotional vulnerability. See Worksheets 7-2 and 7-3.

Worksheet 7-2   ABC PLEASE Inventory of Current Emotional Vulnerabilities

Use this worksheet to take an inventory of the current state of your ABC PLEASE skills.

	In Balance (Yes/No)	What do I do to work on this part of ABC PLEASE?	What does it look like when I am not taking care of this ABC PLEASE skill?
Accumulate Positives			
Build Mastery			
Cope Ahead			
Treat Physical Illness			
Lather Rinse Repeat/ Limit Screen Time			
Balanced Eating			
Avoid Mood-Altering Substances			
Balanced Sleep			
Exercise			

Worksheet 7-3 Weekly ABC PLEASE Tracking Sheet

PRACTICE

Use this worksheet to track your ABC PLEASE skills for a week. Write down what you are doing in each of the boxes to keep balance. If you have many areas out of balance, pick two specific areas to focus on and find balance.

	Monday	Tuesday	Wednesday	Thursday	Friday	Saturday	Sunday
A							
B							
C							
P							
L							
E							
A							
S							
E							

After you have completed your inventory and spent some time tracking your PLEASE skills, think about which ones have the greatest impact on your mood. Worksheets 7-4 and 7-5 help you reflect on these skills.

Worksheet 7-4   ABC PLEASE Skills Weekly Tracking Reflections

Which of the ABC PLEASE skills are most challenging for you to practice? Is there anything you can do to improve these skills? What red flags can you look out for to signal yourself to be mindful of balancing your ABC PLEASE skills? Remember, you have a lot of control over your ABC PLEASE skills, so be creative.

_____

_____

_____

_____

_____

_____

Worksheet 7-5   PLEASE Skills Red Flags and Reflection

Take a moment to reflect on your ABC PLEASE skills and some of the red flags that can alert you that your skills are out of balance. Identifying your red flags will help you decrease your emotional vulnerabilities and attend to areas that will help you feel more able to manage strong emotions that come your way.

_____

_____

_____

_____

_____

_____

Remember that taking care of your ABC PLEASE skills creates a sturdy foundation and makes you less vulnerable to intense emotions and challenges that you face.

SUN WAVE NO NOT

Mindfulness is the core skill of DBT and while it has its own module, mindfulness skills show up in all of the modules. Mindfulness of your current emotion using the SUN WAVE NO NOT method is in the Emotion Regulation module. As discussed, it is critically important to notice and label your emotions.

If you find this challenging, the SUN WAVE NO NOT method will help you decode what you are feeling. As you become more skillful, you will find yourself using your distress tolerance crisis survival skills (covered in Chapter 9) less and increasingly using this skill to ride the wave of your strong emotions. This acronym is a step-by-step guide to being mindful of your current emotion:

>> **Sensations:** Since all emotions have associated body sensations, your body can tell you a lot about how you are feeling. You may have heard people say they have butterflies in their stomach when they feel nervous or anxious. Take a moment and scan the sensations in your body. Start at your head and face and move down to your toes. Look around for different sensations. Do you feel tightness or tension in your jaw or the muscles in your face? Tightness in your chest or shoulders? A fluttering or sinking feeling in your stomach? Tears in your eyes?

>> **Urges:** Recall that one of the three functions of emotions is to motivate actions. It therefore makes sense that all emotions have associated urges. For example, when you feel sad, you may have the urge to cry, curl up, or isolate. When you are anxious, you may have the urge to escape, run, freeze, or fight. When you feel shame, it is common to have the urge to hide and avoid. When you are angry, you may have the urge to yell, throw something, or attack. Other people may isolate or cry when they are angry. People don't always have the same action urges, but they tend to be similar.

>> **Name the emotion:** Once you have identified your body sensations and your urges, you should have enough information to name or label your emotion. In most situations, you will notice that once you can name your emotion, the intensity of the emotion will go down a bit. Being able to name your emotion is the first step in making a little space between you and your experience of an emotion. Using this skill will help you identify any primary emotions that are hidden beneath secondary emotions.

>> **WAVE:** The next step in being mindful of your current emotion is to learn to ride out the experience. We learn from the model of emotion that you experience primary emotions like a wave. The experience starts at a low intensity, increases until it peeks like the crest of a wave, and then decreases like a wave arriving at the shoreline. To effectively ride the wave, you use the observe and describe mindfulness skills discussed in Chapter 6.

Go back to your sensations and urges and practice observing and describing them — that is, noticing and labeling them non-judgmentally. You will notice that when you mindfully observe and describe your emotions, you will slowly return to your emotional baseline. Stick with your sensations and use phrases like, "I notice the urge to. . ." and "I notice the sensation of. . ." These types of mindful observations help you create some separation from yourself and what you are feeling and protect you from unintendedly enhancing the very emotions you want to decrease.

If you notice that this process is boring, you are on the right track! Without judgments and editorials, you will stay with your primary emotions. Remember, primary emotions only last around 90 seconds.

NO NOT: The final part of this skill is NO NOT. NO NOT gives you some specific tips to help you effectively ride the WAVE.

>> **NO:** No suppressing your emotions and no enhancing your emotions when you are mindfully riding the wave. This means do not do things that make your emotions more intense. Judgments and invalidation are the most effective way of enhancing the very emotions that you are working to decrease. Our brains often add to the emotion, for instance by remembering similar situations, which fuels the fire. Notice this and steer back to just this emotion. Remember to not suppress your emotions by telling yourself not to feel what you are feeling or by practicing other forms of avoidance.

>> **NOT:** As you are riding the wave, you need to remind yourself that you are NOT your emotions and that these emotions will NOT last forever. We tell ourselves that we are emotions when we say things like *I am sad* or *I am anxious*. When you use this type of wording, you are essentially telling yourself that you are a sad person and that is a fixed state that cannot change.

We know that emotions come and go. When you talk to yourself, you need to make sure that is clear. It may be a small semantic change, yet it goes a long way. So, what should you say? You want to use phases like *I feel sad* or *I feel depressed.* This signals the brain that this is an experience that will change, which is important to remember when you are experiencing strong and challenging emotions. Remember, emotions do not last forever, and sometimes, you will have to remind yourself of this fact. Use Worksheet 7-6 to practice SUN WAVE NO NOT.

Worksheet 7-6   SUN WAVE NO NOT

Use this worksheet to practice SUN WAVE NO NOT. For an added challenge, use this worksheet when you feel anger and see if anger is a secondary emotion.

Sensations (what do you notice in your body?):

_____

_____

_____

Urges (what do you feel like doing?):

_____

_____

_____

(continued)

Name the emotion (using the list of primary emotions, what makes sense with the data you gathered in your S and U)

_____

_____

_____

Ride the WAVE (observe and describe your sensations and urges using *I notice* statements).

_____

_____

_____

Remember: NO suppressing/NO enhancing. You are NOT your emotions and emotions will NOT last forever. Did you notice any slips into your NOs and NOTs?

_____

_____

_____

Changing how you feel with opposite action

While the ABC PLEASE skills support your long-term emotion regulation and reduce your emotional vulnerabilities, *opposite action* is a powerful emotion regulation skill that can change how you feel in the moment. Remember that sometimes your emotions do not fit the situation, because you are feeling them too deeply or they are lasting too long, causing you to be ineffective, or getting in the way of your goals. Earlier in this chapter, we labeled these emotions as unjustified. The urges that are associated with unjustified emotions often lead to ineffective behaviors. Opposite action helps you change your emotions and get back on track.

Opposite action can seem easy, but it is a skill that takes a lot of willingness, which sometimes can be hard to generate. The great thing about opposite action is that the payoff is big and the effects last a lot longer than distress tolerance crisis survival skills. Opposite action also teaches your brain new information — you can behave independently of what your emotion is urging you to do!

To understand how opposite action works, consider this example. You are anxious to go to work because you must tell your boss that you cannot pick up an extra shift, and you are afraid she will be angry or disappointed. You skip dinner the night before and go to bed. The next morning, you wake up anxious, feeling like you cannot get out of bed. You decide you will not go to work. It makes sense that you are anxious, as setting limits is very challenging for you. However, while your anxiety makes sense, the intensity of your anxiety is too high (your boss has never been angry at you or your co-workers who have not been able to work extra shifts) and the long-term consequences of not showing up to work will make your situation much worse. Moreover, you don't know if your boss will be angry, but it feels like she will be. You can see that following your urge to stay in bed and avoid the issue will be very ineffective. This skill asks you to act opposite to this urge 110 percent.

The following steps lead you through practicing opposite action:

1. **Identify and name your primary emotion(s).** You can use the SUN WAVE NO NOT skill to do this.

    I am afraid that my boss will yell at me and no longer like me, which will mean I will get bad shifts moving forward. I am ashamed that I can't go to work and take care of this like other people do.

2. **Check the facts and determine whether the emotion is justified or unjustified.**

    It makes sense that I am anxious, as I have difficulty setting limits and saying no to people. The intensity of my anxiety does not make sense, and it has been going on for too long. My boss has never yelled at me, I have gotten good reviews, and she is normally understanding in such cases.

3. **Ask yourself: What is my action urge? What do I want to do or not do as a result of how I feel right now?**

    I want to stay in bed, not show up to work, never go back to work, and turn my phone off so no one at work can reach me.

4. **Connect with your wise mind (see Chapter 6) — both how you feel about the situation as well as the fact of the situation — and ask yourself whether acting on these urges is effective for your long- and short-term goals.**

    Acting on these urges is not effective. I like my job and have a good relationship with my boss, who has been very supportive and has not been angry when my co-workers have not been able to pick up extra shifts. I have also changed jobs a lot and it is important on my resume to show that I can hold a job longer than a few months.

5. **If your emotion or its intensity is unjustified and it is ineffective to act on your current urges, identify some ways you can act opposite or very differently than your current ineffective urges.**

    I will get up, shower, turn my phone on, and go to work.

6. **Act opposite 110 percent.** Go further than just acting opposite. Throw yourself in and take risks that help ensure that you will be doing something very different than the ineffective urges. The further you can go, the more powerful the impact on how you feel.

    I will get up, shower, get dressed, make a cope ahead plan, turn my phone on, and text my manager asking to find a time to check in about her request during today's shift. I will also tell one friend about my plan.

7. **Continue the process of acting opposite until your urges and emotions decrease.**

    I will continue to act confident, assertive, and review my plan until I am able to speak to my boss. I will keep my phone on.

REMEMBER This skill takes a lot of willingness, but the payoff is big. Once you have practiced opposite action a few times and felt the benefit, it will be easier to practice moving forward because the positive results will reinforce your efforts. Worksheet 7-8 helps you practice opposite action. This skill can lead to strong feelings of mastery and increased motivation to keep using it. Try Worksheet 7-7 to identify your challenging emotions.

Worksheet 7-7 Identifying My Challenging Emotions and Associated Action Urges that Get Me Stuck

PRACTICE Use this worksheet to identify common problematic or challenging emotions and their urges that have negative impacts on your life when you act on them. Most people have common emotions that get them stuck over and over and those common emotions have common behaviors associated with them.

Common Challenging Unjustified Emotions	Action Urges that Get in My Way When I Act on Them	Negative Consequences as a Result of Acting on These Urges

PRACTICE

Worksheet 7-8   Practicing Opposite Action

Use this worksheet to practice your opposite action skill. Work your way through all seven steps.

Step 1: Identify and name your primary emotion(s).

_____

_____

_____

Step 2: Check the facts and determine whether the emotion is justified or unjustified.

_____

_____

_____

Step 3: What is your action urge? What do you want to do or not do as a result of how you feel right now?

_____

_____

_____

Step 4: Connect with your wise mind — both how you feel about the situation as well as the facts of the situation. Is acting on these urges effective for your long- and short-term goals?

_____

_____

_____

(continued)

Worksheet 7-8 *(continued)*

Step 5: If your emotion or its intensity is unjustified and it is ineffective to act on your current urges, identify some ways you could act opposite or very differently than your current ineffective urges.

_____

_____

_____

Step 6: Act opposite 110 percent.

_____

_____

_____

Step 7: Continue the process of acting opposite until these urges and emotions decrease.

_____

_____

_____

Chapter **8**

Interpersonal Effectiveness

I nterpersonal effectiveness is another one of the four main skills modules of DBT. This chapter helps you learn and practice skills to support effective relationships. Relationships are complicated and as a result, can prompt intense emotions that can lead you to engage in behaviors that get in the way and are detrimental to your long-term goals.

In this chapter, you review and practice interpersonal skills to be more effective at asking for things and getting what you want, saying no and maintaining your self-respect, nurturing important relationships, as well as managing interpersonal anger. Learning to use your interpersonal effectiveness skills will help you build and maintain healthy relationships.

WARNING

Interpersonal effectiveness skills are some of the most challenging to practice. What makes these skills so challenging is that you are using them with other people, and you cannot always accurately predict other people's behaviors, responses, or vulnerabilities. In addition, exchanges between people are frequently fast-paced. You need to stay mindful and remember your skills, even when the pace is fast and the emotions are strong.

Understanding What Gets in the Way of Your Relationships

Relationships are complicated, and there are multiple things that can make you ineffective. There are several factors that can negatively impact how effective we are with other people. Remember, these factors are universal and affect all of us, whether we are doing DBT or not (see Worksheet 8-1).

Here are some obstacles that get in the way of being interpersonally effective:

>> **You don't have the skills you need:** Remember that DBT is a skills deficit model, so people coming to DBT have skill deficits in certain areas. DBT teaches these skills.

>> **You don't know what you want:** Being effective is challenging when you don't know what you want. It is important to remember that knowing what you do *not* want is not the same as knowing what you *do* want. If you have a desired outcome in mind, it is important to take time and consider what you do want out of an interaction. Your emotions can be one of the biggest barriers to knowing what you want.

>> **Your emotions get in the way:** Emotions are one of the biggest culprits to interpersonal effectiveness. I am sure you have heard someone say, "I can't believe I did or said that." That is usually a result of our emotions getting in the way because you were driven by your powerful emotions and were not able to stop and think. If you are an emotionally sensitive person, you are at a higher risk for emotions getting in the way of your relationships and you may have been told that you are "too much" by people in your life.

>> **You forget your long-term goals for your short-term goals:** Strong emotions can make it difficult to hold on to longer-term goals. Strong emotions typically drive you toward short-term gratification and doing what feels best in the moment, even if it isn't best for you in the long run. Forgetting your long-term goals can make it hard to maintain long-term relationships.

>> **Other people get in the way:** There are times when other people are more powerful than you, no matter how effective you are. This could be a boss, coach, teacher, parent, police officer, or someone else. You may start out being effective but when you realize the other person is more powerful than you, you may quickly become less effective.

>> **Your thoughts and beliefs get in the way:** Your thoughts profoundly impact your behaviors. Certain types of thoughts can get in the way of your relationships. Thoughts around being underserving or believing you know how other people feel about you and being driven to convince people you are right can negatively impact your relationships and make them hard to keep in the long term.

Worksheet 8-1   Things That Get in the Way of My Interpersonal Effectiveness

Now that you have reviewed the list, complete this worksheet. Take a few minutes to write down some examples in any areas you have noticed recently.

Factors That Get in the Way	Examples/Reflections
I don't have the skills	
I don't know what I want	
My emotions get in the way	
I forget my long-term goals	
Other people get in my way	
Thoughts and beliefs get in my way	

Mastering DEAR MAN Skills

This module highlights three different areas of effectiveness and each area has an associated skill. The three areas are as follows:

>> Objective effectiveness, or learning to effectively get what you want

>> Relationship effectiveness, or nurturing the relationship and the other person's emotional experiences

>> Self-respect effectiveness, which involves learning to uphold and maintain your self-respect in relationships

All three of these areas of effectiveness are important in relationships and at times, we have to prioritize one area over another. This chapter teaches you the DEAR MAN skills, which will help you with objective effectiveness, the GIVE skill, which will teach you the critical skill of validation so that you can nurture your relationships and practice understanding yours and the other person's emotional experience, and finally the FAST skill, which teaches you to maintain your self-respect in relationships.

DEAR MAN is your objective effectiveness skill. In other words, DEAR MAN helps you effectively ask for what you want. Many times people who come to DBT struggle to effectively ask for what they want and have a hard time hearing the answer no. This is often due to strong emotions getting in the way. In many cases, what you are asking for may be quite reasonable, and it may be the way that you ask that makes it hard for the other person to say yes. The DEAR MAN skill helps you slow down, clarify exactly what you want, and ask for it in an effective way that maintains your relationship with the other person. However, just because you ask effectively does not mean that they will say yes every time. It does increase your odds significantly, though. If they do say no, you will have asked in a way that did not damage the relationship.

This section breaks down the DEAR MAN skill. Notice that this is one of the longer acronyms in DBT. It helps you slow down and really think about what you want and how you will ask for it. DEAR MAN is very hard to do when you are in emotion mind, so make sure you are in a wise mind when developing your DEAR MAN skill (see Worksheets 8-2 and 8-3).

>> **Describe:** This may feel different to you. Start your DEAR MAN by describing a few facts of the situation. Think about bringing the other person to the table and describing only the facts that you both agree with.

   Example: I have worked here for one year, and I have taken four days off. I worked both Christmas and New Year's Day.

>> **Express:** Many people start their asks with how they feel. In DBT, you express how you feel after you describe the facts. Now you share how you feel about the situation. Remember you are only sharing how you feel. Do not make assumptions about how the other person feels.

   Example: I have not spent time with my extended family in some time, I miss them, and want to see them. I am sad that I have missed several holidays with my family.

>> **Assert:** Now you ask for what you want. The most effective asserts are when you ask the person a yes or no question. Figure out exactly what you want and ask for it. Don't use phrases like "It would be nice." or "I would appreciate it if. . ." Be direct and assertive in asking for what you want.

   Example: Can I take five days off at the beginning of the next pay period?

>> **Reinforce:** Reinforce is one of the most important parts of the DEAR MAN skill. The reinforce is a unique part of this acronym and can really increase the effectiveness of your ask. The easiest way to understand the reinforce is to think about what is in it for the other person to say yes to your request. This means you need to think about your request from the other person's perspective. Remember, it has to be what is important to them, not to you. Why should they say yes to you?

WARNING

A common mistake is to say to the person, "If you say yes, it will make me happy." That is a weak reinforce because it is more about you.

   Example: I know it is difficult to find coverage and Annie has agreed to cover my shifts because she is not on the schedule that week. I will also meet with her a few days before I leave and brief her on my projects. I will also introduce her to the clients she will be working with so that they also understand the plan and coverage while I am away.

» **Mindful:** Mindful begins more of what are called the style points of DEAR MAN. It is easy to get off track when you are asking for something. Mindful reminds you to stay focused on your assert. If you get off topic or are led off topic intentionally or unintentionally by the other person, stay mindful and gently return to your assert statement.

Example: I hear that a number of people have asked for time off in the past and not provided coverage. At the same time, I rarely ask for time off and have my week completely covered. Can I please take the time off that we discussed?

» **Appear confident:** How you deliver your DEAR MAN makes a big difference. Consider your eye contact, speech volume, and body language. Writing out your DEAR MAN and even rehearsing it can also increase your confidence.

» **Negotiate:** This final part of the DEAR MAN is the negotiate. We like to say that you always want to have a negotiate in your back pocket. Hearing no can be very challenging. The minute some people hear no, their emotions escalate, and it becomes hard to stay effective in the conversation. Planning out a negotiate can expose you to the thoughts and feelings that may arise should you hear no. Think about hearing no — what feelings arise? Now think about a negotiate that will allow you to stay engaged with your ask. For every DEAR MAN, you should have at least one negotiate.

Example: I hear that the first week of the next pay period will not work because two other people have requested that week off. Would the first week of the following pay period work, as that will give me enough time to find coverage and make new plans with my family?

Worksheet 8-2   DEAR MAN Reflection

Looking at the DEAR MAN acronym, which areas come easier to you? Which parts are more challenging and why? Write your reflections here.

_____

_____

_____

_____

_____

_____

_____

Worksheet 8-3   DEAR MAN Worksheet

Use this worksheet to practice writing out a DEAR MAN for an upcoming ask you are planning to make. At the end, review your DEAR MAN and reflect on how using DEAR MAN may be similar or different from how you would typically make this ask.

Describe:

_____

_____

_____

_____

Express:

_____

_____

_____

_____

Assert:

_____

_____

_____

_____

Reinforce:

_____

_____

_____

Mindful:

_____

_____

_____

Appear Confident:

_____

_____

_____

Negotiate:

_____

_____

Reflections:

_____

_____

_____

_____

The Art of Validation

Validation is the key to nurturing relationships and helping other people feel like you are curious and understand their experience given who they are. On the surface, validation can seem simple; however, you will learn it is really an art. Validation can also be challenging because, as you learned with DEAR MAN, strong emotions and the fast pace of a conversation can be barriers to effective validation.

On the most basic level, validation is finding the wisdom in the other person's emotional experience given who they are. It is important to realize that you may not feel the same way, because you don't experience emotions like they do. Yet you still need to recognize that, given who they are, their emotions make sense.

REMEMBER

Remember, validation is not agreement or an endorsement of a behavior; it is simply a recognition of someone's feelings. When your emotions are strong, it can be challenging to validate someone else's emotions. This is because strong emotions make it difficult for you to consider perspectives other than you own, which is a key part of validation.

Many people who come to DBT have experienced a lot of invalidation of their emotions — being told they are too sensitive, making a big deal out of something, should let it go, or "get over it." For emotionally sensitive people, this kind of invalidation can make validating others very challenging.

We are often asked, how do you know if your validation is right or working? Validation has some powerful emotion regulation properties. When you get validation right, two things often happen:

>> The intensity of the conversation, both the volume and the speed, tend to slow down when the person feels understood.

>> The other person begins to talk more and share more about their experiences and how they feel. They may even ask for help.

SELF-VALIDATION

Due to chronic invalidation, people who come to DBT also have trouble validating their own emotions and often spend a good deal of time self-invaliding, which leads to escalating challenging emotions, difficulty identifying how you feel, and ineffective problem solving. It often leads to extended states of misery. Self-validation is a critical step in understanding your emotions, labeling them, and making sense of them. Learning to validate yourself helps you navigate and recover from the invalidating world around you. Self-validation skills are the same skills you use to validate others. When you are self-validating, you are reminding yourself that how you feel makes sense. This will help you understand yourself better, think about what you need, effectively problem-solve, and choose the most effective skills for the situation.

There are also two indicators you can look for to let you know that your attempt at validation was not effective or did not land well for the other person:

>> They tell you in an often loud and direct way how much you do not understand or how unhelpful you are.

>> They shut down, get quiet, and the communication or conversation stops. The good news is that you can always try again and see if you can get it right.

REMEMBER

There are a couple of important things to remember. Validation is one hundred percent about the other person. You are not sharing your experience when you are validating someone else. Validation should always be tentative. You are not telling the other person how they feel. Think of it more like you are checking in to see if you are understanding their experience. Finally, if the other person tells you that you are not right or do not understand, you agree with them, step back, and get curious again.

Validation from others helps you feel more understood and can be used to better understand painful experiences from the past. It is also critical for maintaining relationships. When you're coming to DBT, validation helps you feel more understood and helps you learn how to self-validate. See Worksheets 8-4 and 8-5.

Building blocks of validation

The most common question we get is, "So how do I validate and what do I say?" This section shares six different ways to validate. What makes validation challenging and an art form is that we cannot provide a script, as then it does not sound genuine.

WARNING

When you begin to practice validation, it may feel clunky or robotic. It may be hard to find your words or you may even be accused of speaking weird or like a therapist. Hang in there and acknowledge that you do probably sound different because you are trying something new to better understand the other person. If you are honest about trying a new skill, most people will cut you some slack.

Here are Linehan's six levels or ways to validate:

>> **Pay attention:** Give someone your full attention. Put your phone or computer down, maintain eye contact, nod so they know you are following along, or ask clarifying (non-leading) questions. All of these behaviors let the other person know that you are curious and interested about their experience and how they feel.

>> **Reflect back:** When you reflect back, you are letting the other person know that you want to make sure you understand how they feel. Don't reflect back the obvious, like if they are yelling then saying something like, "You are angry." Reflect back with curiosity, "You are angry because you were left off the email and missed the meeting, did I get that right?" You can also reflect back by saying something like, "You seem really sad right now." Again, what works in one situation and with one person may not work with another person or a different situation. With practice, you will get a sense of how to reflect back effectively to the people in your life.

>> **Read minds:** This type of validation is what we call "high risk, high reward." When you get this validation right, it has a very positive impact. When it does not land, you need to have an apology ready in your back pocket. The reading minds validation is understanding how someone feels by paying attention to their body language and their behavior instead of relying on a conversation. This type of validation feels great, because sometimes it is nice to know that someone understands how you feel without you having to talk about it. If you get it wrong, you can always apologize and then go back to being curious using your pay attention validation.

>> **Understand:** This type of validation involves understanding how the person feels given their history. This validation is a great opportunity to make sense of your emotions. For example you could say, "It makes sense that you are anxious about your meeting with your boss, because the last meeting you had he cut your hours."

A note about the word "understand." In general, we advise against using the phrase "I understand." While your intentions are good, when you use this phrase, you violate the principle that validation is one hundred percent about the other person by introducing how *you* feel or understand. Furthermore, you must be mindful that you really do understand exactly how the other person feels by having had the same experience and by experiencing emotions exactly as they do. As you get more skilled at validation, there may be some people in your life who are okay with using the phrase "I understand." We advise that you use it as sparingly as possible. Instead, try "It makes sense you would feel that way," "Or I can see that you feel. . .".

Acknowledge the valid: This is also a great clarifying type of validation. By acknowledging what is valid, you are letting the other person know that their experience makes sense because it is a common experience shared by many people. For example, it makes sense that you are anxious about starting a new job, because first days can be stressful as people learn to navigate a new job.

>> **Show equality/radical genuineness:** This type of validation relies less on words and more on behaviors. With this type of validation, you want to be your authentic self in recognizing another person's experience. This can look like tearing up when someone shares that they are sad, handing someone a tissue, giving someone a hug, and joining in someone excitement when they are very happy. Be mindful not to hijack their experience, but use yourself to show them that you understand their experience.

Worksheet 8-4   Understanding the Types of Validation

Match the examples with the type of validation. You'll find the answers at the end of this chapter.

A. Pay attention	1. It makes sense that you are anxious about your first job interview; many people are also anxious in interviews, especially when they have not done very many before.
B. Reflect back	2. Without asking any questions you say, "tough day?"
C. Read minds	3. You seem really frustrated with the situation.
D. Understand	4. Putting your phone down, making eye contact, and asking clarifying questions.
E. Acknowledge the valid	5. Handing someone a tissue when they are about to cry.
F. Show equality/radical genuineness	6. It makes sense that you are worried about dating; your last relationship ended in such a painful way.

Worksheet 8-5   Practicing Validation

Now that you have learned the different types of validation, take a few minutes to come up with examples of each type. Think of current experiences with people in your life and use the worksheet to practice how you could be validating.

Pay attention:

_____

_____

_____

Reflect back:

_____

_____

_____

Read minds:

_____

_____

_____

Understand:

_____

_____

_____

Acknowledge the valid:

_____

_____

_____

Show equality/radical genuineness:

_____

_____

_____

_____

Validating when you disagree

One of the hardest parts of validation is validating when you disagree with the other person. While this is hard, it is a critical skill to master to support your relationships.

REMEMBER

Remember that validation has nothing to do with agreement; it has to do with acknowledging the validity in how the other person feels. When you think about it this way, validating when you disagree should feel more manageable.

EXAMPLE

Consider this example. Your friend applies for a job that they are not qualified for. When they do not get the job, they get really angry and tell you all about how unfair it is. The challenge here is that you agree that they should not have gotten the job because they are not qualified. The relationship is important, and your friend is really upset. Now is not the time to explain why they did not get it. How do you validate them? Here are some ways you could validate their response:

>> I hear how upset and disappointed you are that you didn't get the job.

>> I hear that it feels really unfair to you that you did not get the job.

>> It seems like you really wanted this job.

Notice that in each of the examples, you are not agreeing that it's unfair. You are simply acknowledging the possible emotions. Once the other person is more regulated, you can talk with them about some of the reasons you think they might not have gotten the job, which could be helpful feedback for the future. However, right now emotion mind is running too high to have a reasonable or rational conversation with them. See Worksheet 8-6.

Worksheet 8-6   Validating When You Disagree

Think of a recent example when you disagreed with someone in your life and could have used validation to nurture the relationship and help them feel understood even though you strongly disagreed with what they were saying. Write down the example and come up with three different validating statements.

Describe the situation:

_____

_____

_____

_____

_____

Write down three different validating statements despite your disagreement:

_____

_____

_____

_____

_____

_____

_____

_____

Communicating with GIVE Skills

Marsha Linehan put the skill of validation in the GIVE acronym. You have already learned about the most challenging part of this acronym, which is the V for validate. The other parts are more style pointers to enhance your effectiveness. Let's break down the GIVE skill:

>> **Gentle:** You must be gentle and tentative when you are validating someone. Be kind and stay away from a harsh tone, attacks, or threats. Stay curious and avoid judgments.

>> **Interested (Act):** Try to be interested in what the other person is sharing. If you are not truly interested, you must act interested. Ask open ended questions and be curious. Think about taking a learning stance — lean in and don't interrupt.

>> **Validate:** Use your six types of validation. Check in with yourself as well and be connected with your own feelings as you pay attention to how the other person feels.

>> **Easy manner:** This part of GIVE can be deceivingly hard, especially if validation is a new skill for you. Take a breath and validate with ease. Stay away from intensity, which can be challenging when you are working hard to find the right words. Stay with it, smile, and use light humor as long as it is not invalidating.

GIVE helps you add some style to the six types of validation reviewed earlier in this chapter. Sometimes, you will just validate using your GIVE skill; other times you will combine validation with the other interpersonal effectiveness skills we teach throughout this chapter. See Worksheet 8-7.

Worksheet 8-7   Practicing GIVE Skills

Use this template to write out in detail an example of validating someone in your life using GIVE. Remember, you will use the GIVE skill when validating someone who you agree or disagree with.

Gentle:

_____

_____

_____

_____

Interested:

_____

_____

_____

_____

Validate:

_____

_____

_____

_____

_____

Easy Manner:

_____

_____

_____

_____

_____

_____

Staying True to Yourself with FAST Skills

The third skill in this chapter is the FAST skill. The FAST skill is about maintaining your self-respect. This skill helps you leave situations feeling like, no matter the outcome, you behaved according to your values about how you want to treat other people and with a sense of integrity. This skill is very effective for saying no or setting a personal limit. For some, setting limits alone can be hard. For others, the way that they set limits often damages relationships and gets in the way of short- and long-term goals. See Worksheet 8-8.

Effective FAST skills should not be used in an emotion mind.

WARNING   Let's break down the FAST acronym:

>> **Fair:** It is critical to be fair to you and the other person. This means taking some time to look at the situation from your and the other person's perspectives. This is nearly impossible to do when you are in an emotion mind. Find a balanced position where you can see both perspectives and figure out what is fair for both of you. It is a slower process to set fair limits.

>> **No apologies:** You need to apologize when you have hurt someone or done something that has crossed your values. You do not need to apologize for setting a limit, even if it is difficult for the other person to tolerate. Over-apologizing degrades your self-respect and dilutes the meaning of apologies when you really need to use one. Stay confident, even if it is hard for you to say no.

>> **Stick to your values:** Connect with your own values and what is important to you when you are in a wise mind. Don't sell yourself short, but stand behind your own morals and values. You may need to spend some time thinking about your own interpersonal and general values and morals. It is good to clarify your values from time to time.

>> **Truthful:** You must own your limit as yours. Do not hide behind ideas like "everyone is doing it," "is it appropriate or inappropriate," or make excuses. Acknowledge that this is your limit and your reasoning.

Worksheet 8-8   Practicing FAST Skills

Use this worksheet to plan a limit/to say no someone in the next couple weeks. Describe the situation. Who do you need to set this limit with and what are the barriers that you can anticipate? Can you problem-solve any barriers that may arise?

Situation:

_____

_____

_____

_____

_____

Barriers to setting your limit:

_____

_____

_____

_____

Ways to address or plan for the barriers:

_____

_____

_____

_____

Fair:

_____

_____

_____

_____

No apologies:

_____

_____

_____

_____

Stick to your values:

_____

_____

_____

_____

Truthful:

_____

_____

_____

_____

_____

Combining GIVE and FAST Skills

Although we teach these interpersonal effectiveness skills separately, the more you practice them, the more you will find that they work well in combination. We have found that FAST is most effective when you combine it with GIVE. People hear limits and hard news better when they feel like you have spent some time thinking about and acknowledging how it will make them feel.

The key is to link these skills with the word *and* or *at the same time.* This type of linking creates a dialectical balance in which both your validation and your limit are equally important. The biggest mistake people make is to use the word *but.* When you do this, you negate the validation that came first, so be mindful not to fall into that trap.

Here are some examples of how you can put the GIVE and FAST skills together:

» I see that you are really angry that I won't continue this conversation, and I will not continue to be yelled at because it is not good for either of us in the long run.

» I know you really wanted to get the promotion and, at the same time, you have come late to work four times in the last month, so I am not able to promote you.

» I know you just learned that a bunch of your friends are getting together, and we already made plans with the family, which we need to keep.

Notice that you begin with validation using GIVE and then you set your limit using your FAST skill. See Worksheet 8-9.

Worksheet 8-9 Combining Your GIVE and FAST Skills

Use the example you used from Worksheet 8-8 and add three ways to validate before you set limits using FAST.

Write your FAST (from Worksheet 8-8)

_____

_____

_____

_____

GIVE +and/at the same time FAST

_____

_____

_____

_____

GIVE +and/at the same time FAST

_____

_____

_____

_____

GIVE +and/at the same time FAST

_____

_____

_____

_____

Managing Interpersonal Anger with THINK Skills

Now that you have learned how to effectively ask for something, validate other people's feelings, set limits, and stand up for your self-respect, this section explains how to manage one of the emotions that can cause significant problems in your relationships — anger. Many people who come to DBT struggle with managing anger. In fact, difficulty managing anger is one of the symptoms of Borderline Personality Disorder (BPD), which is one of the primary disorders that DBT was developed to treat. There are two ways people often struggle with anger:

>> Some people struggle managing surges of anger and lash out, yell, or scream, say hurtful things, make threats, get physically aggressive, or break things.

>> Other people suppress anger so much that they have trouble accessing it and tend to turn anger inward against themselves.

Both approaches are problematic and both interfere with healthy relationships. Chapter 7 covers more about anger and skills that you can use to regulate it.

One of the skills that will help you with interpersonal anger is practicing *perspective taking* and considering another person's point of view in times when you feel like they have wronged you. To do this, you are challenged to shift from an emotion mind to a wise mind (we talk about DBT states of mind and the wise mind in Chapter 6). The THINK skill helps you do this when you are in a disagreement or are feeling angry at someone. The THINK skill takes you through this process step by step. See Worksheet 8-10.

Let's break down the THINK skill:

>> **Think:** Think about the situation from the other person's perspective. Don't let go of your position, but open your mind and get curious about where they are coming from. Put yourself in the other person's shoes. Why might they be thinking and feeling the way they are?

>> **Have empathy:** Now focus on what they might be thinking and feeling. Use your validation skills to make sense of how they are feeling if you are having difficulty understanding them. Don't share your validation, just think about it, and pay attention to how you feel when you consider their perspective. Consider if they are feeling hurt, worried about losing something or someone, or feeling misunderstood or undervalued.

>> **Interpretations:** When you get angry, you are prone to make negative assumptions about the other person and their intentions. These negative assumptions tend to fuel your anger. Notice those assumptions and make a list of other possible benign interpretations of their behavior. Think about positive reasons why the person is holding that position or engaged in that behavior.

>> **Notice:** Spend some time noticing how the other person is trying to improve or do things better in their life. Consider times they have been kind, helpful, or supportive. Ask yourself if there is something going on or something they are currently struggling with that may be contributing to their behavior.

>> **Kindness:** Remember to be kind and take a gentle and kind approach as you consider all of the steps of the THINK skill. Lead with kindness in your interactions with the person.

Worksheet 8-10   Managing Interpersonal Anger and Conflict with the THINK Skill

Use this worksheet to decrease your anger at someone in your life.

Briefly describe a recent or current conflict.

_____

_____

_____

_____

Next, try to shift your anger and open your mind to more perspectives by completing each step of the THINK skill.

Think:

_____

_____

_____

_____

Have empathy:

_____

_____

_____

_____

(continued)

Worksheet 8-10 *(continued)*

Interpretations:

_____

_____

_____

_____

_____

_____

Notice:

_____

_____

_____

_____

Kindness:

_____

_____

_____

_____

TIP

Remember that these skills take practice! You may find it helpful to practice these skills during times of lower emotion and with relationships that are less emotionally charged. The worksheets in this chapter should be a resource that you use often. Remember that you can find blank worksheets online as well (at www.dummies.com/go/dbtworkbookfd). You will find the structure of the worksheets helpful as you are learning. The more you practice, the more confident you will become. Over time, you will rely less on the worksheets to plan ahead. Remember that one of the ways to reduce emotional vulnerabilities (discussed in Chapter 7) is to cope ahead. Remember your DEAR MAN, GIVE, FAST, and THINK skills when planning for interactions that you know will be challenging.

Worksheet 8-4   Answers

A4: Pay attention: Putting your phone down, making eye contact, and asking clarifying questions.

B3: Reflect back: You seem really frustrated with the situation.

C2: Read minds: Without asking any questions you say, "tough day?"

D6: Understand: It makes sense that you are worried about dating; your last relationship ended in such a painful way.

E1: Acknowledge the valid: It makes sense that you are anxious about your first job interview; many people are also anxious in interviews, especially when they have not done very many before.

F5: Show equality/radical genuineness: Handing someone a tissue when they are about to cry.

IN THIS CHAPTER

» **Using crisis survival skills**

» **Making decisions using pros and cons**

» **Identifying barriers to acceptance**

» **Working to accept reality**

» **Creating your own crisis kit**

Chapter **9**

Distress Tolerance

D
istress tolerance is one of the four skills modules of DBT. This module is divided into two parts — crisis survival skills and accepting reality skills. Many of these skills may seem familiar or fall into the category of "coping skills" that you have learned in other treatments. This module provides many skills, and they are organized into a number of acronyms to help you remember. This module is all about acceptance skills, so none of these skills will provide long-term solutions to problems that you are facing. The goal of acceptance skills is three-pronged — help you get through the moment without making things worse, help you decrease the intensity of your emotions in the short-term, or help you with an ongoing practice of accepting the reality that is in front of you.

What Is Distress Tolerance?

Distress is part of all of our lives and the intensity of our distress can wax and wane throughout our lifetimes. People who are emotionally sensitive may experience more distress, as they feel things more deeply and for a longer time than others. Sometimes, a high level of distress may make it difficult to solve problems or use skills that can provide longer-term relief. Although it does not cause all distress, one big contributor to distress is being unable to accept reality, especially if it's unwelcome.

The first half of the distress tolerance skills are *crisis survival skills*. These skills are designed to be the first part of a chain that helps you when your emotions are too high. You use a longer-term emotion regulation skill or engage in problem solving. To put it another way, these skills help take the edge off so that you do not make a situation worse by doing, not doing, saying, or not saying something that will have long-term undesirable consequences. When you are deep in your *emotion mind* (engaging with the world around you based on how you feel and not what you know — see Chapter 6 for more), your first step in finding balance is to try a couple distress tolerance crisis survival skills.

WARNING

Distress tolerance skills should be the first in a series of skills that you use. Distress tolerance skills are not designed to solve problems, only to decrease the intensity of strong emotions. Moreover, they only are built to work while you are using them. Once you stop using the skill, the problem that caused your distress is still there. If you find that you are feeling like DBT skills are not working, check in with yourself and make sure you are not relying too heavily on these skills because too much time using only crisis survival skills will leave you exhausted and frustrated.

You will learn that there is a fine line between crisis survival skills and avoidance. There are two very important things to remember about these skills:

>> You must use them deliberately and with intention.

>> They must be used in a time limited way (typically no more than a few hours).

Employing Crisis Survival Skills

People often ask us how to remember the specific situations in which they should use crisis survival skills. Here are some situations:

>> You are experiencing very strong emotions and feel that the only way to make them decrease or end is to engage in one of your maladaptive target behaviors that will make you feel better in the moment but make things more difficult in the long run.

>> You are experiencing deep emotional pain that feels too much to manage and it just won't end.

>> You feel overwhelmed and want to give up and avoid but have to meet an obligation or deadline.

>> You want to solve a problem right now and you must wait hours or until the next day to address the problem or figure out a solution.

>> You are experiencing panic or overwhelm and are having a hard time doing anything.

REMEMBER

Crisis survival skills can be very helpful, and they must be the first of a chain of skills that you use to address a problem at hand. You can think about these skills as helping you regulate so that you can then use other skills to address the problem in front of you.

The DBT crisis survival skills are organized into a number of acronyms to help you remember them, including ACCEPTS, IMPROVE, TIPP, and STOP. The following sections look at each of these skills in detail. At the end of this chapter, we ask you to create some crisis survival skills and build your own crisis kit.

Distracting with ACCEPTS and IMPROVE

Distraction skills tend to be the most familiar to people when they come to DBT and are a way of taking your mind off a problem that is causing you distress. Many people have learned coping skills to distract from how they are feeling. Some of these skills may be very familiar, while other ones may be newer ways to distract. Our goal is to enhance the number of skills you can use to get through difficult movements and give the skills structure/organization to make using them more accessible.

The first skill is the ACCEPTS skill:

>> **Activities:** Activities are the most common distraction skill and one that you probably have used before. Your task is to throw yourself into an activity to shift your attention from what is upsetting you. You can do any activity! Popular activities are going for a walk, watching a TV show, calling a friend, playing a game, coloring, doing a puzzle, playing an instrument, cleaning, or doing a craft. Some activities are more or less distracting and take more effort, so pay attention to which activities are most distracting when you are feeling specific emotions.

>> **Contributing:** This is one of our favorite distractions! The act of distracting yourself requires you to shift your attention from what is upsetting you to doing something for someone else. This skill has a bonus, as contribution often leads to positive emotions and makes us feel good because we are doing something for someone else. It is great to contribute in your life, and when you use it for distraction, think about small things that you can do. Some examples are to call someone who you know would appreciate talking to you, writing someone a letter or email of appreciation, doing a chore or task around the house, or even going to a coffee shop and paying for the coffee of the person behind you.

>> **Comparisons:** You must be careful when using this skill, as many people who come to DBT use comparisons as a way to invalidate themselves. You essentially compare yourself to a less skillful version of yourself. For example, six months ago I would not have been able to manage this type of disappointment and been able to get up and go to work the next day. You are highlighting that you have come some way and become more skillful in order to be using this skill effectively.

>> **Emotions:** Here, you are distracting yourself by creating a different emotion. For instance, you may feel sad and choose to watch a YouTube video of puppies, which elicits feeling of love and joy. Other ideas are watching things that make you feel fear like horror movies or comedies that make you laugh. Activities like skipping, dancing, and laughing can also powerfully change how you feel. Before you use emotions, make sure that you self-validate how you are feeling in the beginning, so that this process does not feel invalidating.

>> **Pushing away:** As with the contribution skill, you need to be mindful about how you practice pushing away. This skill is best used to temporarily distract yourself and push away what is painful or avoid an unsolvable problem because it feels intolerable, and you can't cope with it in the moment. The critical part of this skill is that you must have a plan to come back to it. Write down the problem or painful emotional experience and set a time when you will return to it and address it skillfully. Some people imagine building a wall or fence between them and the problem or even leaving the situation, taking a break, and returning later. If you do not return to the problem, you have simply practiced avoidance, which is not a skillful distraction.

>> **Thoughts:** This skill allows you to distract yourself by engaging your mind in thinking tasks. These are cognitive tasks to engage your mind. Think about skills like counting backward by

seven, doing crossword puzzles or Sudoku, or picking a category and using the alphabet to come up with something that starts with each letter. We even worked with someone who solved math problems as a distraction.

>> **Sensations:** Here you are using sensations to distract yourself. Consider sensations like cold showers or holding ice while it melts, warm showers or using a heating pad, eating something very sour or spicy like a fireball candy, and then focusing on the sensations that are produced. Taste and smell can also be powerful distractors.

Worksheet 9-1 helps you practice the Wise Mind ACCEPTS skill.

Worksheet 9-1 My Wise Mind ACCEPTS

While you may not use each one of these skills, fill in the boxes with some examples of how you could practice each of these skills.

Activity	My Practice
Contribution	
Comparison	
Emotions	
Pushing Away	
Thoughts	
Sensations	

The next set of distraction skills is called IMPROVE the moment. If you cannot solve the problem in front of you, you can try your best to shift how you feel. Again, you are looking to improve the moment, not solve the problem. Here is how you can do it:

>> **Imagery:** The practice of imagery is imagining a situation different than the one you are in. The idea is to change the situation in your mind or use your mind to imagine a different situation that helps change how you feel. If you are in distress, it may be helpful to imagine a situation that brings you a feeling of calm and peace. Think about images that are pleasant and calming. All of us have our own unique places we can go in our minds that bring us a sense of calm. Using all of your senses in your imagery will make it more powerful.

>> **Meaning:** Meaning is a powerful skill and one in which you make meaning of difficult and painful things that have happened or are happening to you. Making meaning of your pain and suffering helps you find purpose in the experience. This is a very challenging skill and very powerful when you are able to do it. It can also be difficult. Think about the positives in your difficult situation. Marsha Linehan describes this as "making lemonade out of lemons." One common way we recommend is by highlighting that the stressful situation is an opportunity to practice strengthening DBT skills!

>> **Prayer:** This can be religious-based or not. For people who are religious, they can find peace in prayer and asking for help from a higher power. For many, prayer helps see them through a crisis. For some it is not about religion, but about asking for help from something bigger than us that can also provide relief in times of suffering.

>> **Relaxation:** In a crisis, both your body and mind can be tense. Relaxation skills can help shift your attention toward relaxation. A nice way to practice this is to inhale and tense up a muscle group and then on your exhale focus on relaxing those muscles. There are many guided relaxation exercises online.

>> **One thing in the moment:** This is where mindfulness is incorporated into the distress tolerance module. When you are in distress and feeling overwhelmed, you can really suffer. This skill involves tolerating your distress by taking it one task at a time. Doing one thing in the moment will help you focus and do that one thing to the fullest. Make a list, complete one task at a time, and you will feel more settled and be able to slow down. Stay focused on the present and bring your mind back when it catapults you into the future. Some people find it helpful to say to themselves, "I am doing the most I can right now in this moment (to finish these tasks, deal with this issue, and so on.)."

>> **Vacation:** Sometimes you need a break. Long vacations are great but for this skill, we want you to take a mini-vacation. You can do this with imagery, or you can plan an activity. Consider taking a 30-minute walk, watching a show or two, driving to a hiking trail and going on a short hike or walk on the beach, closing your office door and taking a short nap, or even going on an overnight trip somewhere. Be mindful that when you use this skill, it might create problems if your vacation gets in the way of deadlines or other commitments.

>> **Encouragement:** This is a very challenging and powerful skill and one that you should work on outside of the moment of crisis or distress, so you have it ready when you need to use it. You might find this skill particularly challenging as many people who come to DBT struggle to encourage themselves. This practice asks you to find a way to encourage yourself during difficult moments. You have to find a way to talk to yourself that you will believe. Think about things like, "I'll get through this, I am more skillful now," "This is challenging, and I've got this," or "Stay steady and keep going." Research shows that people who effectively encourage themselves increase their ability to perform the task they are doing. Use Worksheet 9-2 to develop your own encouraging statements. Worksheet 9-3 helps you work on the IMPROVE skill.

PRACTICE

Worksheet 9-2   Diving into Encouragement

Use this worksheet to come up with three different encouraging statements that you could use and practice them over the next couple months.

1.

_____

_____

_____

_____

2.

_____

_____

_____

_____

3.

_____

_____

_____

_____

Worksheet 9-3   IMPROVE the Moment

PRACTICE

Fill in the boxes in this worksheet with some examples of how you could practice each of these skills.

Activity	My Thoughts
Imagery	
Meaning	
Prayer	
Relaxation	
One thing in the moment	
Vacation	
Encouragement	

Calming yourself with self-soothing

Self-soothing skills (see Worksheet 9-4) involve calming yourself using your five senses. This is also a distraction skill that works by shifting your attention using sight, hearing, smell, taste, and touch. Many of these skills may overlap with your other distraction skills. The acronyms are to help you remember your skillful options. Use your sense of

>> **Sight:** Look at something that will distract you and capture your attention. Look at the clouds moving in the sky or people in a park or at the mall, go on a walk and look at nature, or look at pictures that bring you joy.

>> **Hearing:** Listen to your favorite music, try to find the quietest sound in the room, listen to sounds of nature, or listen to the traffic outside.

>> **Smell:** Light a scented candle, smell essential oils, put on your favorite lotion or soap, or smell a food that you like.

>> **Taste:** Mindfully eat something you enjoy, savor it in your mouth and focus on the taste. Drink something you enjoy and focus on the taste.

>> **Touch:** Think about soothing textures and items. Pet your dog or cat, hug a stuffed animal, wrap yourself up in a soothing blanket, or put on comfortable soft soothing clothing. Some people have also found running their fingers over things like Calm Strips can also be soothing.

TIP

Calm Strips are textured sensory stickers, often with a reusable adhesive. Many people find that they help them manage their restless energy.

PRACTICE

Worksheet 9-4   Self-Soothing Skills

Using this worksheet, identify four ways you can practice soothing yourself with each of your five senses.

Sight	1.
	2.
	3.
	4.
Hearing	1.
	2.
	3.
	4.
Smell	1.
	2.
	3.
	4.
Taste	1.
	2.
	3.
	4.
Touch	1.
	2.
	3.
	4.

Taking the edge off with TIPP

The TIPP skill is a different take on how to regulate your distress quickly (see Worksheet 9-5). We get many complaints that distress tolerance skills do not work quickly enough and certainly don't work as quickly as many of the self-destructive behaviors seem to.

This is in fact true. The TIPP skill is DBT's way of using skills to regulate the body. As a result, these skills can reduce your distress much faster than the other crisis survival skills. The TIPP skills work by rapidly changing your body chemistry, which can capture your attention and help you feel more regulated.

TIP

>> **Temperature:** The goal with temperature is to activate your mammalian dive reflex, which is a primitive reflex in your brain that has the ability to slow down your heart rate and calm the fight or flight response that is activated when you get dysregulated. The most effective way to do this is to activate the cold sensors under your eyes.

We teach people how to do this by having them do an ice dive. Fill a bowl with ice and very cold water and dunk your face in it a few times, until you notice that your heart rate has slowed, and you begin to feel calmer. While this works powerfully on your physiology, most people also experience a break in their thought loop, as it becomes hard to focus on anything except the cold on your face.

This is the fasted working skill in DBT; however, the downside is that it is not very portable! To mimic it in a smaller way outside of your kitchen, you can put ice (or a cold compress or frozen peas!) on your cheeks and jaw bone while you bend over or lean over and splash cold water on your face.

>> **Intense exercise:** This acts on your physiology in the opposite way of temperature. While temperature down-regulates and slows your heart rate, intensive exercise increases your heart rate. Try exercise like running stairs, holding planks, running sprints, or doing wall sits for longer periods of time. Do the exercise as quickly as you can (getting to 50-70% of your maximum heart rate) for 20 minutes, if you can, and then breathe and let your physiology slow back down.

WARNING

If you have a heart condition or any other medical condition in which quick changes to your heart rate are dangerous, please consult your doctor before using the TIPP skill.

>> **Paced breathing:** Many types of breathwork can also slow down your physiology. Paced breathing is a great breathing exercise for managing anxiety, because it's a quick cue to your parasympathetic nervous system to engage. The key to paced breathing is that your exhale has to be longer than your inhale. Breath in slowly for five seconds and then exhale slowly for eight. Actually, you can use any length of inhale and exhale, but you must make sure your exhale is longer.

>> **Paired muscle relaxation (PMR):** This is another skill that slows down your physiology and is also a great practice during mindful attention. The most effective way to do this is to pair your muscle tension and relaxation with your inhale and exhale.

It can look like this. Inhale and contract the muscles in your face, and hold. On your exhale, relax the muscles in your face. Inhale and contract your shoulders, drawing them up to your ears and holding them. On your exhale, relax them down your back. Continue to contract one muscle group at a time all the way down to your toes — then start back up your body again one muscle group at a time until you get back to your face. Some people find it's also helpful to think "calm" or "relax" as they release the tension in the muscle group.

Worksheet 9-5   It's Time to Use TIPP

Using this worksheet, think about situations or emotions in which you could use each of these TIPP skills to manage strong emotions.

Temperature	
Intense Exercise	
Paced Breathing	
Paired Muscle Relaxation	

Remember that some of the TIPP skills increase heart rate and are what we call *activating*, while other TIPP skills are focused on calming your physiology.

Slowing down with STOP

When people are dysregulated, they have a tendency to move too quickly, whether it is saying things they don't mean, trying to solve problems, or making decisions that are emotion minded. Not being able to slow down and find your wise mind in times of distress can ultimately damage relationships and cause long-term problems. The STOP skill will help you in these moments.

>> **Stop:** Stop! Don't give into your urge to do or say something. Pause and find your balance. Don't yell, don't send that text or email, or give in to your urge to do a target behavior. Picture a stop sign or even say the word "stop" to yourself.

» **Take a step back:** Make some space between you and the situation. This could be going to another room, outside, or pausing and taking two deep breaths.

» **Observe:** Take a moment to observe how you are feeling. Use your SUN WAVE NO NOT skills discussed in Chapter 7. Pay attention to your emotions. Now observe what is going on around you. What are the other people thinking and feeling? Articulate all of this to yourself.

» **Proceed mindfully:** Once you have completed the first three steps, consider the situation. Think about your goals and the outcome you are looking for. Ask your wise mind what you should do next. Make a deliberate decision about what comes next and what will be in line with your long-term goals.

The STOP skill helps you gain control of impulsive and emotion-minded behaviors. Use Worksheet 9-6 to think of a time that you could have used the STOP skill to slow down and gain control of impulsive behaviors.

Worksheet 9-6   Practicing the STOP Skill

PRACTICE

Think of a time recently when your emotion mind got the best of you and you said or did something you wish you hadn't. Think about how you could have used the STOP skill to slow down and curb your impulsive behaviors.

Describe the situation:

_____

_____

_____

_____

Now apply it to the STOP skill. Be as detailed as possible when you think about what you could have done more skillfully.

Stop:

_____

_____

_____

(continued)

Take a step back:

_____

_____

_____

Observe:

_____

_____

_____

Proceed mindfully:

_____

_____

_____

Making wise decisions with pros and cons

The final crisis survival skill involves the process of listing pros and cons. Like a few of the other crisis survival skills, you must complete this one in a wise mind so that you can reference it when you are dysregulated as a way of accessing your own wise-minded wisdom and decisions.

This skill is a practice of evaluating the short-term and long-term advantages and disadvantages of engaging in a specific behavior or making a decision. You are likely familiar with pros and cons lists, but the DBT pros and cons are a little different. DBT pros and cons are more comprehensive, as we ask you to create a four-way grid evaluating the pros and cons.

REMEMBER

If you are evaluating whether to engage in a specific behavior in DBT, we ask you to evaluate the *pros and cons of doing the behavior* and the *pros and cons of not doing the behavior.*

The most effective way to list your pros and cons is to fill up all the boxes as best you can. You might consider even sleeping on it and looking at it the next day to see if you are missing anything. Once you have filled all the boxes with your pros and cons, go back and circle the long-term pros and cons. This is not about the number of pros and cons you have in each box, but about looking at the long-term impact and making a decision based on what is in your best interest in the long term See Worksheet 9-7.

When listing your pros and cons, follow these steps.

1. **Articulate the behavior or decision that you are evaluating.**

2. **List the pros and cons in each of the four quadrants.**

3. **Circle the pros and cons that are consistent with your long-term goals.**

4. **Evaluate and make your decision.**

EXAMPLE

Pros of staying at this job	Cons of staying at this job
Pros of getting a new job	Cons of getting a new job
Pros of continuing to use weed to regulate	Cons of using weed to regulate
Pros of using DBT skills	Cons of using DBT skills

Worksheet 9-7   Practicing My Pros and Cons

Using this worksheet, think about an upcoming decision that you need to make and complete your pos and cons. Remember to do your best to include as many pros and cons you can think of. Once you are finished, go back and circle the long-term pros and cons in each box.

Pros of Making the Decision	Cons of Making the Decision

Pros of Not Making the Decision	Cons of Not Making the Decision

Accepting Reality

The distress tolerance module is the only module that is divided into two parts. The previous section reviewed the crisis survival skills and this section now covers the accepting reality skills. These skills are some of the most challenging skills in DBT, *and* they have the most robust impact on changing the way you regulate your emotions and navigate your life.

In this section, you learn and practice three skills that help you accept the reality in front of you — radical acceptance, turning the mind, and willingness and willfulness.

Practicing radical acceptance

Learning and practicing radical acceptance can truly be life changing. Accepting a reality that you do not like is hard and most people fight against it. The problem with fighting a reality that you don't like is that the reality does not change, and you are left suffering.

To deal with and problem-solve difficult situations, you must first accept them. It is not uncommon for the process of acceptance to be substantially more difficult than the problem solving that follows.

REMEMBER

You must remember these four things when you are practicing radical acceptance. Radical acceptance is:

>> Acceptance of THIS moment and the reality in front of you right NOW.

>> NOT agreement or liking something.

>> A practice OVER and OVER, because it is very easy to slip out of acceptance.

>> Not necessarily how something should be; it is how something IS RIGHT NOW.

There are absolutely going to be some things that are easier and other things that are harder to accept. Accepting that a loved one has hurt you, that you have a chronic illness, that you were passed over for a position that you deserved, that you have lost someone in your life — these are all situations that require acceptance.

TIP

Radical acceptance is whole heartedly opening yourself up to the reality in front of you. It involves looking at whatever is there with open eyes and accepting it with your heart and soul. People often ask how to tell if they are in acceptance. Many people say that when you find a place of acceptance, you feel a sense of calm, like the struggle around something has softened. They know this has happened, it cannot change, and the suffering and rumination disappears. While suffering dissipates, sadness may arise.

When teaching this skill, we remind people that with acceptance often comes loss. When you accept something that you have been struggling with, you often have to let go of something that you expected or hoped would be different. With that comes a healthy sadness that needs to be validated and soothed.

WARNING

It can be easy to fall into accepting a future that has not happened. This is what we call *resignation*. Most people have struggled with resignation at some point when they try to accept a future that has not happened and say things like, "I just have to accept that I will never get promoted" or "It's okay that I will never get married." While many people think anticipating a bleak outcome will make them feel better should it happen, it simply does not work that way. Using your Cope Ahead skill from ABC PLEASE (see Chapter 7) is a much more effective way to plan for a future you are worried about.

REMEMBER

While resignation is a very passive process, radical acceptance is a very active process of working with your attention. Radical acceptance is a practice you must do over and over again. The more challenging the thing you must accept, the more you will move in and out of acceptance before it sticks. Use Worksheet 9-8 to contemplate your barriers to radical acceptance and Worksheet 9-9 to help practice radical acceptance.

PRACTICE

Worksheet 9-8   My Barriers to Radical Acceptance

What makes it hard for you to practice radical acceptance? What thoughts and behaviors get in the way? Use this worksheet to identify what gets in the way of you accepting reality. Think about your thoughts and behaviors that make it hard to accept.

Thoughts:

_____

_____

_____

_____

_____

Behaviors:

_____

_____

_____

_____

_____

Worksheet 9-9   Practicing Radical Acceptance

PRACTICE

Use this worksheet to think of a situation that you are having a hard time accepting. Sit somewhere quiet and work on whole heartedly practicing radical acceptance. Write down the situation and your observations before and after your practice.

The situation I need to accept:

_____

_____

_____

_____

Observations of non-acceptance:

_____

_____

_____

_____

How did I practice radical acceptance:

_____

_____

_____

(continued)

_____

_____

Observations after the practice:

_____

_____

_____

_____

_____

_____

Turning the mind

It would be great if you could practice radical acceptance once and everything would be hunky-dory, but as discussed, most times it is something you have to do over and over again. The skill that you use to move back into acceptance when you fall out is called the *turning the mind* skill. You will use your mindfulness skills from Chapter 6 to notice when you are in non-acceptance and work to *turn your mind* and attention back toward acceptance.

Follow these steps to practice turning your mind back to acceptance when you fall out of it.

1. **Use mindfulness to notice when you are in non-acceptance.**

2. **Sit upright in an open position and rest your hands palms up to signal to your body that you are open to new information and change.**

3. **Make a commitment to shift your attention back toward acceptance.**

REMEMBER

Turning the mind is not acceptance, it is a shift in your attention and a commitment back to focusing on your practice of acceptance.

TWO PRACTICES TO HELP YOU WITH ACCEPTANCE

There two physical acts that you can practice, both of which communicate to your brain to take a more accepting and willing approach — Willing Hands and Half-Smile.

Willing Hands

1. Take a few breaths.

2. Uncurl your hands.

3. Rest your hands gently on your lap, palms up if you are seated, or by your side if you are standing.

4. Relax your fingers and allow your hands to slightly curve as if you are receiving something.

Half-Smile

1. Take a few breaths, relaxing the muscles in your face.

2. Focus your attention on the small muscles at the corners of your mouth.

3. Allow the corners of your mouth to turn up just slightly. For many people, their half-smile is undetectable by other people.

4. Some people find it helpful to then think about smiling with their eyes.

Understanding willingness and willfulness

Willingness and willfulness are directly related to acceptance. There are the behavioral manifestations of both states.

>> *Willingness* is the intentional practice of seeing and accepting things as they are. Willingness is an openness and attitude of participating in the world as it is and all that comes with it — the ease and the challenge.

>> *Willfulness* is the opposite of willingness. Willfulness is the refusal to accept reality and participate in life as it is. Willfulness is a painful non-accepting state that is driven from a deep-seated sense of fear or threat that something important to you is at risk. Willfulness is driven by the emotion-mind and you must be careful because it can be contagious and polarizing. Use Worksheet 9-10 to identify your own willfulness.

REMEMBER

One of the first steps to catching your non–acceptance can be recognizing when you are in a state of willfulness. Do not judge your willfulness because you got there honestly, just notice it. From there, you can use your turning the mind skill and then work on radical acceptance.

Signs of willfulness:

>> Digging your heals in and doing the opposite of what needs to be done

>> Needing to control everything

>> Giving up

>> Solving problems that are not yours to solve

>> Refusing to see other points of view

Worksheet 9-10   Signs of My Willfulness

Use this worksheet to check off the willful behaviors that you relate to. Next to the box, write how they show up for you.

❑ Doing the opposite of what needs to be done

_____

_____

❑ Needing to control everything

_____

_____

❑ Giving up

_____

_____

❑ Solving problems that are not mine to solve

_____

_____

❑ Refusing to see other's points of view

_____

_____

❑ Feeling physical tension (clenched fists, clenched jaw, squinting eyes, and so on)

_____

_____

❑ Other: _____

_____

_____

❑ Other: _____

_____

_____

❑ Other: _____

_____

_____

Putting It All Together: Your Own Crisis Kit

As you have learned, distress tolerance is a large two-part module. Because there are so many skills, it can be helpful to sort through and group together the skills you prefer to use when you are in distress. We recommend that you create a list that you can keep on your phone or create a box, bag, or basket with items that you can reference when you are in crisis or high distress.

When you are learning DBT and in distress, it can be difficult to remember which skills you should use and how to use them. Creating your own crisis kit will give you a place to look and skills to choose from, so you do not have to flip through this chapter and try to determine which skills could be helpful. Your crisis kit should have at least ten different skills and any items you need to practice the skill. Crisis kits are a wonderful way to support learning and practicing the distress tolerance skills.

Use Worksheet 9-11 to check off which skills you will put in your kit and provide details about the materials you will include or notes you will write to yourself about how to use the skill.

For example, you could check off pros and cons and include a note that you will make a copy of your pros and cons about ending a relationship and put it in your box or take a picture of it on your phone. You may check off activities and then make a list of the specific activities you want to do when you are using the activities skill from the ACCEPTS skill. It may be helpful to also think about which skills will be helpful in certain emotions. Be as specific as possible so that you will have a comprehensive list to build your crisis kit.

As an example, consider the contents of Kirsten's (a fictional alcoholic) crisis kit, which she uses when she feels an urge to drink:

>> Knitting (A in ACCEPTS)

>> Scented Candle (smell self-sooth)

>> Crossword puzzles (T in ACCEPTS)

>> Card with "I can do hard things" written on it (E in IMPROVE)

>> Pros and cons list for drinking

>> Putty (S in ACCEPTS)

>> Pictures of her dog, cat, and friends (Sight self-sooth)

>> Lavender oil (Smell self-sooth)

>> Note card with three-minute intense exercise sequences (I in TIPP)

>> Picture of ice cubes (T in TIPP)

>> My favorite minds (Taste self-sooth)

>> Compassion prayer written on a card (P in IMPROVE)

PRACTICE

Worksheet 9-11   Components of My Crisis Kit

ACCEPTS

❑ Activities _____

❑ Contribution _____

❑ Comparisons _____

❑ Emotions _____

❑ Pushing Away _____

❑ Thoughts _____

❑ Sensations _____

IMPROVE

❑ Imagery _____

❑ Meaning _____

❑ Prayer _____

❑ Relaxation _____

❑ One Thing in the Moment _____

❑ Vacation _____

❑ Encouragement _____

Self-Sooth

❑ Vision _____

(continued)

Worksheet 9-11 *(continued)*

❑ Hearing _____

❑ Smell _____

❑ Taste _____

❑ Touch _____

TIPP

❑ Temperature _____

❑ Intense Exercise _____

❑ Paced Breathing _____

❑ Progressive Muscle Relaxation _____

❑ Pros and Cons _____

❑ STOP _____

❑ Turning the Mind _____

❑ Willing Hands _____

❑ Half-Smile _____

I will keep my crisis kit _____

_____

IN THIS CHAPTER

» **Understanding the purpose of the middle path**

» **Discovering dialectics**

» **Being mindful of the middle path**

» **Fostering dependency and forcing autonomy**

» **Searching for synthesis**

Chapter **10**

Walking the Middle Path

When Drs. Alec Miller and Jill Rathus modified DBT to create DBT for adolescents, they added a module called *Walking the Middle Path.* This additional module focuses on skills for adolescents and their parents or caregivers and looks at common dialectical dilemmas. This module has two main skills — parenting dialectical dilemmas and behaviorism. Chapter 5 covers behaviorism, and this chapter covers parenting dialectical dilemmas.

In teaching dialectical dilemmas, this set of skills will also help you better understand the concept of dialectics. It may help you, as an adult, understand some of your parent's behaviors as well as your own. Understanding dialectics can help you see the world — your own behaviors and other's — in a more complex and nuanced way. This chapter introduces the concept of dialectics and digs into the three common dialectical dilemmas that parents and adolescents face: fostering dependency and forcing autonomy, being too loose and too strict, making light of problem adolescent behaviors, and making too much of typical adolescent behaviors.

What Is the Middle Path?

The middle path skills are a set of skills to help people, particularly parents, learn to find balance between two or more opposing viewpoints. The goals of these skills are to help parents become more aware of areas in which they may get stuck in all-or-nothing, emotion-minded parenting, notice when they feel divided and judgmental of one another when co-parenting, recognize when they swing back and forth from extreme reactions to their child's behavior, remind them that these are common difficulties, that they are not alone, and fundamentally improve communication between adolescents and parents.

WARNING

Dialectics is a good tool to use when you feel stuck or polarized and can't seem to move forward when you're trying to understand behavior or solve a problem. One of the biggest challenges of dialectical thinking and behaving is that it is very hard to do it in an emotion mind! Before you can be dialectical, you must regulate your emotions!

Dialectics vs compromises

Dr. Marsha Linehan, who developed DBT, did not come up with the theory of dialectics. In fact, the theory of dialectics dates back to the 19th century. According to the Oxford English Dictionary, *dialectics* is defined as "the art of investigating or discussing the truths of opinions and the inquiry into metaphysical contradictions and their solutions." So, what does this mean? Dialectics is about two or more opposing truths existing at the same time.

When you are thinking dialectically, you are looking for multiple truths, even if they seem to be opposites. You are searching for the wisdom or what makes sense in each truth. A helpful question to ask yourself when you are trying to think dialectically is, *what am I missing?* This question helps open your mind to other possibilities.

There are many dialectics in DBT, and the foundational dialectic is acceptance and change. This dialectic makes DBT different from CBT. Both are behavioral treatments that help people change their behavior, but DBT does this through using dialectical interventions and teaching acceptance skills (mindfulness and distress tolerance) and change skills (emotion regulation and interpersonal effectiveness).

In DBT, we accept that you are doing the best you can *and* recognize that in order to change in ways that bring you closer to your goals, you have to do better, try harder, and be more motivated to change. Both are true at any given time! An even more extreme example is that when you are thinking dialectically, you may consider the opposite of the truth not a lie, but instead another truth!

How is dialectical thinking different from a compromise? When you are thinking dialectically, you are looking for a synthesis of the multiple truths that you discover. That is, you take my perspective and yours and give them equal value. You consider what makes sense about each of these perspectives and is there a way to synthesize them into a new perspective or a way to move forward?

What can be a bit confusing about these skills is that a synthesis is not necessarily the middle; it may incorporate more of one perspective or solution than the other. In the process, you demonstrate value in all perspectives as you look for a way forward. The key is not to get stuck in the absolute.

In general, a compromise is easier and faster to find than a synthesis. A compromise is much more about making an agreement in which both sides make concessions, meaning you only need to negotiate. You can come to a quick solution that often does not really address the fundamental problem or people's thoughts and feelings about it. A *synthesis*, on the other hand, focuses on the thoughts and feelings behind the problem and then looks for a solution. It tends to take much more time.

Dialectics is about two or more opposing truths existing at the same time.

Letting go of either/or and welcoming both/and

As you have learned, dialectics is about multiple truths existing at the same time, even if they appear to be opposing ideas. When you think dialectically, you use words such as *and* and *at the same time*, and each truth holds equal weight. Thus, by definition, you are moving away from *either/or* and toward *both/and* statements. When you are thinking dialectically, you are using words such as *and, at the same time, sometimes*, and *rarely* and staying away from absolute words such as *always, never, every*, and *but*. You are holding two or more ideas together.

Dialectical thinking will help you find solutions and see perspectives when you find yourself stuck. It is a powerful way to manage difficult situations and make wise-minded decisions. Dialectical thinking will also help you navigate conflict and maintain healthy relationships. Try Worksheet 10-1 to get started. Worksheet 10-2 can help you practice your dialectical thinking.

Worksheet 10-1   Generating Dialectical Thinking Using AND

Use this worksheet to provide a true opposing statement and make the statement dialectical. You can add your own at the end of the table as well.

Example: I want to do things differently	AND	I am afraid of change
I am doing the best I can	AND	
I am angry at them	AND	
I feel like I failed	AND	
I want to be alone	AND	
I disappointed them	AND	
I need to be alone	AND	
I disagree with you	AND	
I want to be independent	AND	

(continued)

Worksheet 10-1 *(continued)*

Example: I want to do things differently	AND	I am afraid of change
I feel anxious	AND	
I don't want to do this	AND	
I understand your perspective	AND	
I feel hopeful things will change	AND	
	AND	
	AND	
	AND	
	AND	

Worksheet 10-2   Practicing Dialectical Thinking

Use the situations described on this worksheet to practice your dialectical thinking.

1. Think about an interaction that you found challenging in the last week or so in which you were certain about the other person's intentions or motives. Generate three different possible reasons for why they behaved the way they did. Remember, you are searching for what you may have missed. If you know the person well, think about who they are, their past, and their values, all of which can influence their position.

_____

_____

_____

_____

_____

2. You are about to cross the street at a crosswalk when a driver honks his horn and does not stop, speeding across the cross walk. You get scared and immediately think, this stuff always happens to me, and that person doesn't care to follow the law. How can you think about this more dialectically? Think about your feelings and the reasons why this may have happened.

_____

_____

_____

_____

_____

3. A friend doesn't call to follow up and see how you are doing after you shared you were having a difficult week. You immediately conclude that they don't care. What is a more dialectical way to look at this?

_____

_____

_____

_____

_____

(continued)

4. Think about something you want to change. This could be doing more or less of something. When we want to make a change, it is easy to get absolute about it, for example, I will go to the gym every day, stop eating sugar completely, and never go off my meal plan. Make a plan to change a behavior and do so dialectically. Stay away from *always* and *never* and be dialectal in your plan.

_____

_____

_____

_____

_____

_____

Middle Path Dialectical Dilemmas

Now that you understand that dialectics involves investigating the truths of opinions and contradictions and their solutions, you can jump into the middle path dialectical dilemmas. As stated, there are many dialectical dilemmas in DBT and in your life. In addition, there are three specific ones that parents with adolescents in DBT seem to be very challenged by:

>> Fostering dependency and forcing autonomy

>> Too loose and too strict

>> Making light of problem adolescent behaviors and making too much of typical adolescent behaviors

These three dialectics are highlighted by Drs. Miller and Rathus in their adolescent treatment manual. Remember, when you name the dilemmas, you are noting the poles or extremes of the dialectics. While these dilemmas are not uncommon to parents whose children are *not* receiving DBT, they tend to be more challenging for parents who have adolescents who struggle with emotion regulation and self-destructive behaviors.

REMEMBER

Highlighting these dilemmas provides a tool for parents to better understand their own positions. If you are co-parenting, it can help you better understand another perspective and find compassion and respect even when you disagree. Understanding and practicing dialectical thinking when parenting will improve communication and nurture your relationship with your child.

When it comes to making parenting decisions, there can be strong emotions involved, which makes people more vulnerable to emotion mind, absolute thinking, which can interfere with wise-minded decisions, and make dialectical thinking a challenge. As you learn about these dialectical dilemmas, keep in mind that there is no absolute answer, but one specific to each situation. Each time you are faced with one of these dilemmas, work to find synthesis, search for as many perspectives and truths as possible, and then make a decision. Sometimes, the solution may land in the middle, other times it may be more toward the poles. Landing on an extreme is a warning sign that you may be missing important information.

Fostering dependency and forcing autonomy

This dialectic involves striving to bring awareness and find synthesis and balance between *fostering dependence,* or doing too much for your child so that they do not learn the skills they need to be independent, and *forcing autonomy,* or pushing them to be independent before they have the skills to do so effectively. When children are young, they are fully dependent on their parents and, over time, they learn the skills to be independent. In general, the model of teaching skills is when children are young, parents do many things and solve problems for them; as they get older, parents do tasks alongside them to teach and support the development of a new skill. Once the child grasps the skill, they usually send the message that they know how to do the task and push to do it independently, thereby demonstrating mastery over the task. At that point, parents can confidently withdraw assistance.

When you have a child with deficits in certain areas, it is easy to fall into the habit of doing things for them and unintentionally *fostering dependence.* While this may be done with good intentions, it interrupts the stage of the child learning skills to do the task independently. It is important to remember that, if you are noticing you have done this, you have gotten here honestly. Negative reinforcement (see Chapter 5) encourages you to move in and complete the task, after which both you and your child get a sense of relief.

This is a common dilemma for parents of children with significant anxiety or ADHD, when parents may fall into the habit of organizing backpacks, completing homework, managing medications, or doing tasks like ordering at restaurants and making calls for them. Over time, the child does not develop the skills. The adolescent then relies on their parents for tasks that same-age peers can easily complete and skills they need and often want in order to be independent and successful.

It is also easy for parents to find themselves burned out and resentful for over-functioning, and that is when they are at risk for swinging to the other extreme of the dialectic, which is *forcing antonymy.* Without awareness of this dialectic, parents will begin to get frustrated that their adolescent is not learning developmentally appropriate skills. When this happens, they are at risk of rapidly withdrawing their support, expecting the adolescent to have the skills to be independent. We hear things such as, "People their age should be able to do this!" and then parents withdraw support. The consequences are often dreadful, which can then swing parents back over to the other extreme as they return to fostering dependence. When we see this pattern, we immediately get curious about this dialectic.

TIP

The first step out of this difficult dialectic is awareness! Once you catch it, you can step back and work with it. Remember that strong emotions often drive you to the extreme. Take a dialectical approach and return to the steps of teaching skills to foster learning as you work with your adolescent to move toward independence. See Worksheet 10-3.

Worksheet 10-3   Zooming In on Fostering Dependence and Forcing Autonomy

Use this worksheet to identify how you are fostering dependence or forcing autonomy, what emotions drive you to do so, and a more dialectic approach to building skills. Remember each behavior and dialectical approach may be different since you must practice synthesizing multiple factors.

How I am fostering dependency:

_____

_____

_____

_____

Why do I think I do this?

_____

_____

_____

_____

Emotions that I experience that drive me to the poles:

_____

_____

_____

_____

What I will do differently to be more dialectical:

_____

_____

_____

How am I forcing autonomy:

_____

_____

_____

_____

Why do I think I do this?

_____

_____

_____

(continued)

Emotions that I experience that drive me to the poles:

_____

_____

_____

What I will do differently to be more dialectical:

_____

_____

_____

_____

_____

Too loose and too strict

The second dialectical dilemma for parents is being *too loose* on one end and *too strict* on the other extreme. Finding balance between these two is challenging for all parents. It is very easy for fear to drive parents to the extremes on this one. It is important to remember that if you are co-parenting, it is not uncommon for one parent to be generally looser and the other stricter. This has a lot to do with how you grew up and your own temperament. This is not necessarily a bad thing — it is simply important that you are aware and mindful of it and use it to parent effectively. You need to seek to understand one another when conflict arises.

It can be easy to swing back and forth on this dialectic, but keep in mind that you must consider each situation differently, as there will be times you will be looser and times when you will want to be stricter, depending on the situation and your child's behaviors, symptoms, and skills.

When adolescents are engaging in dangerous or problematic behaviors, parents understandably get scared and it is easy to go to the extreme, clamp down, and try to assert control. Sometimes parents go to the extreme when the situation feels out of control, so they try to control the uncontrollable. That is the most extreme place on this dialectic. Parents move into emotion-minded behaviors, taking everything away or laying down excessive punishments, at which point the adolescent has nothing to lose. While the parent may feel a sense of control for a short time, these punishments are often hard to uphold and an adolescent with nothing to lose can be even more dangerous.

When the *too strict* approach doesn't work, it is easy to willfully throw your hands up and swing over to the other side, which will also prove ineffective and scary. Parents can also find themselves stuck on the too loose pole when they are walking on eggshells afraid to set limits or say no for fear it will destabilize their child's behaviors. See Worksheet 10-4.

Worksheet 10-4   How Fear Leads Me to Be Too Loose or Too Strict

Use this worksheet to think about which factors drive you to the extremes on this dialectic.

Times I Am Too Loose	What I Fear

(continued)

Worksheet 10-4 *(continued)*

Times I Am Too Strict	What I Fear

What would happen if I could decrease my fear?

_____

_____

_____

Once I lower my fear, what is a more wise-minded dialectic response to this issue?

_____

_____

_____

Making light of problem behaviors and making too much of typical adolescent behaviors

This is the last of the three middle-path dialectics, and it can be much more complicated than it looks at first glance. Parents need to find a balance between making too much of problematic behaviors or *pathologizing normal adolescent behavior* and making light of problem behaviors or *normalizing pathological* behavior:

>> *Pathologizing normal adolescent behavior* involves assuming a behavior is problematic or pathological, when in fact it's age-appropriate and normal for an adolescent of a certain age.

>> *Normalizing pathological behavior* is assuming a behavior is typical and normal but in actuality, it needs to be addressed because it is impacting the child's functioning.

There are many challenges that emerge during adolescence. Teens must navigate a number of developmental struggles. They are exposed to drugs and alcohol, sex, school achievement and failure, relationships, more competitive sports and activities, employment, crime, social media, and a drive toward independence. All of these tasks come with a surge in hormones and impulsivity that further enhances emotional reactions and consequences for their behaviors.

Parents and caregivers are forced to try to parse out what is typical and what is not. One way to help you sort through this is to consider how their behaviors impact your adolescent's functioning academically, socially, and within your family. Parents may struggle to determine if behaviors such as increased moodiness, conflict with parents, not wanting to be at home, or spending long periods of time in their room are normal or something to be concerned about. It is important to remember that any forms of self-injury, suicidal ideation, or suicidal attempts are not typical and must be addressed immediately. Worksheet 10-5 goes into this distinction in detail.

TIP

Sometimes the same behavior has a different impact on a child based on their temperament and biology. Pay attention to the frequency of the behavior and how it impacts your child's functioning to help you sort out this dialectic. What is typical now, may not have been when you were an adolescent.

EXAMPLE

Where this dialectic becomes more complicated is when normative or typical adolescent behavior is paired with pathological behavior. For example, Graham comes home after school, drops his backpack, looks upset, goes up to his room, slams the door, turns on his music, and doesn't come out for several hours. This is typical, although not very pleasant, adolescent behavior. However, Tanesha, Graham's mom, knows that in the past when Graham did this, he was also self-injuring, exhibiting suicidal behaviors, and refusing to go to school. This is when the behavior becomes much harder to sort out. Does Graham just need some space after a bad day, or is he cutting again and needs an intervention?

The bottom line is that, as your teen becomes more skillful, you have to give them the opportunity to have these situations and be skillful, despite your mind jumping to pathologizing their teen upset. This is where parents need support, because the process of unpairing these behaviors can be very challenging.

Worksheet 10-5 Assessing Typical Adolescent Behaviors

Use this worksheet to identify three behaviors that you want to look at more closely and assess whether they are typical or a source of concern.

Behavior 1:

_____

_____

Is this behavior impacting my child in the following areas:

❑ Academics

❑ Friendships

❑ Family Functioning

❑ Ability to take care of themselves (eat, sleep, bathe, exercise, and so on.)

❑ Exercise/Sports

❑ Enjoy/Participate in Activities They Enjoy

Based on this assessment, the behavior is Typical or a Problem (circle one).

Do I need to do anything to follow up? Yes, No. If yes, what is my plan to follow up?

_____

_____

_____

Behavior 2:

_____

_____

Is this behavior impacting my child in the following areas:

❑ Academics

❑ Friendships

❑ Family Functioning

❑ Ability to take care of themselves (eat, sleep, bathe, exercise, and so on.)

❑ Exercise/Sports

❑ Enjoy/Participate in Activities They Enjoy

Based on this assessment, the behavior is Typical or a Problem (circle one).

Do I need to do anything to follow up? Yes, No. If yes, what is my plan to follow up?

_____

_____

_____

Behavior 3:

_____

_____

Is this behavior impacting my child in the following areas:

❑ Academics

❑ Friendships

❑ Family Functioning

❑ Ability to take care of themselves (eat, sleep, bathe, exercise, and so on.)

❑ Exercise/Sports

❑ Enjoy/Participate in Activities They Enjoy

Based on this assessment, the behavior is Typical or a Problem (circle one).

Do I need to do anything to follow up? Yes, No. If yes, what is my plan to follow up?

_____

_____

_____

Now you can put it all together in Worksheet 10-6.

Worksheet 10-6   Walking the Middle Path

Use all three middle-path dialectal dilemmas to identify an issue, consider which dialectics are in play, where you fall on the dialectic continuum, where you want to be, and how you will get there. Figure 10-1 shows an example of Walking the Middle Path with a teen.

Current parenting issue or decision you need to make:

_____

_____

_____

Circle the dialectics at play:

Fostering Dependence   Forcing Independence

Too Strict   Too Loose

Making Too Much of Typical Behaviors   Making Light of Problem Behaviors

Identify and write the polar positions for your issue or decision. Put an X where you fall. Put a star where you want to be or feel is the most effective.

_____

_____

_____

How will you shift to this new place and what does that look like? What is the synthesis?

_____

_____

_____

_____

Worksheet 10-6   Walking the Middle Path

Use all three middle-path dialectal dilemmas to identify an issue, consider which dialectics are in play, where you fall on the dialectic continuum, where you want to be, and how you will get there.

Current parenting issue or decision you need to make:

> Cullen is not getting up in the morning for high school unless his dad and I go into his room multiple times and tell him to get up. He usually sets an alarm (although he often does it wrong) but then sleeps through it. This has caused him to be late on multiple occasions, park in inappropriate places, where he got a ticket and then later got a detention, as well as miss classes. We end up in shouting matches with him and nothing works.

Circle the dialectics at play:

Fostering Dependence   Forcing Independence

Too Strict   Too Loose

Making Too Much of Typical Behaviors   Making Light of Problem Behaviors

Identify and write the polar positions for your issue or decision. Put an X where you fall. Put a star where you want to be or feel is the most effective.

wake him up every day   allow him to miss school
and pay the consequences
every time he doesn't get up

How will you shift to this new place and what does that look like? What is the synthesis?

> Cullen knows what he needs to do (go to bed earlier, set an alarm properly, make being on time a priority) and these tasks are age appropriate, so allowing Cullen to fail at his age and pay the consequences is a better approach. This will allow him to handle this problem himself or otherwise pay the consequences (fostering independence). His dad and I will watch from the sidelines to see how often it's still happening and let the school know that we are trying to allow him to work through this problem. If he seems unable to navigate getting up in the morning, we will do some problem solving with him and see if teaching him some other strategies helps him get up independently.

FIGURE 10-1:
Walking the
Middle Path
example.

IN THIS CHAPTER

» Recognizing the dialectical dilemmas

» Working through dialectical dilemmas

» Embracing the paradox

Chapter **11**

Digging into Dialectics

A book on DBT would not be complete without a deeper dive into dialectics. At the core of dialectical thinking and living is the idea that not only do you have to recognize and accept that the universe is filled with opposites, but that because of impermanence and constant change, you are accepting a changing you and changing opposites. For example, over the course of our careers, we have seen adolescents stuck in rebellion against parental authority, only to become parents themselves and be stuck on the opposite side of the struggle, wanting their children to listen and conform!

Recognizing the Dialectical Dilemmas

Marsha Linehan, the developer of DBT, considered dialectical thinking as one of the key principles of DBT. She proposed that there were certain *dialectical dilemmas* that people who came to DBT experienced. These dilemmas are behaviors that were adapted as a direct manifestation of the person's biology, their (invalidating) environment, and their skills deficits, in particular a deficit in problem solving when it comes to emotion regulation.

There are two main ways that people deal with an excess of painful and unrelenting emotions. The first is a tendency to bounce between not being able to control emotions and behaviors, and the second is that they work very hard and tend to over control their emotions and behaviors. It might be easy for you to see why loud emotions and behaviors can be dangerous but it is sometimes less obvious that it's also problematic to mask feelings and squash behaviors. By living in either pole, you aren't able to handle the difficulties that bring you into therapy. For example, if you are feeling excessively sad and angry, and you lash out to people instead of using emotion regulation and interpersonal effectiveness skills, you are likely to use self-destructive behaviors and have unsupportive and temporary relationships. If, on the other hand, you hide your emotions and overly control your behavior, you are invalidating your experience, and everyone will think that you are doing just fine.

When she examined what happened to people with emotion regulation problems, Dr. Linehan noted that people who benefited from DBT struggled predominantly in three dimensions and these dimensions appeared to have opposite poles:

>> The first dimension has emotion vulnerability on one pole and self-invalidation on the other pole.

>> The second dimension has active passivity on one pole and apparent competence on the other pole.

>> The third dimension has unrelenting crisis on one pole and inhibited grieving on the other pole.

Let's look at each of these more closely.

Emotional vulnerability vs self-invalidation

Chapter 1 explains that emotional vulnerability is the biological predisposition that makes a person sensitive. This dialectical dilemma occurs when an emotionally sensitive person struggles to balance this emotional sensitivity with a tendency to invalidate their feelings and experiences. So, on the one hand, emotional vulnerability is being sensitive and easily impacted by emotions, and on the other hand, self-invalidation refers to dismissing, rejecting, or minimizing the significance of this very sensitivity. Self-invalidation is often the consequence of childhood invalidation, where the environment rejected private experiences and this, in turn, led to a cycle of mistrusting internal experiences, judging feelings to be wrong, and feeling that one should not feel the way they do.

Active passivity vs apparent competence

Active passivity is when a person relies on others to solve their problems and make important decisions. At its core, this form of passivity is considered active because the person struggling knows that they are struggling. They learn that, by allowing the problems to grow worse, someone will eventually step in and solve the problem for them. Ultimately, they wait for someone else to resolve the problem rather than resolving it themselves. When this happens regularly, they never learn to solve life's problems.

EXAMPLE

For example, let's say that you are applying to college. You know what you have to do — you have to download the application, answer all the questions, and write a personal statement. You know that. To someone asking you what the process is, you would say "I have to download the application, answer the questions, and write a personal statement." Now imagine that you are filled with so much anxiety about the process that you can't even start. Your parents ask you if you have started, and you don't answer. The application is due in a few days, and you haven't started. You avoid and procrastinate, and your parents are worried. You express how impossible the task is, and your parents now start to panic. Eventually, they take over and fill out the application. Both you and your parents feel better. In your passivity, the system rallied around you to get done what needed to be done. In time, you learn that if you leave things until the last minute, someone will step in, and ultimately, even though you appeared to know what to do, you couldn't do it and when you get others to do it, you don't actually learn.

The other side of the dialectic is termed *apparent competence*. This refers to a person's tendency to appear capable and skilled. They are able to "talk-the-talk" by saying the things that show insight, and that they know what to do. However, they struggle to put this apparent knowledge and competence into action. The competence seems accurate and real but the person cannot do what they say. When this happens, it means that you bounce between telling the world that you know what to do but you don't do what needs to be done through active passivity. This then leads to confusion, frustration, and distress in self and others.

Unrelenting crisis vs inhibited grieving

This is the experience of enduring and continuing crises, often in the context of significant skills deficits, leading to maladaptive coping strategies, which in turn lead to further crises. For instance, say that you are very upset and use crisis behavior such as self-injury, drugs, or alcohol to deal with the distress. Say that this then leads to interpersonal conflict with a loved one, which then upsets you further and leads to a further crisis.

The inhibited grieving side of the dilemma is the various ways — whether active or passive — that a person acts to avoid the powerful emotions caused by loss or trauma. This includes active or passive ways that people avoid or escape their emotions, particularly emotions relating to loss or grief. In this dilemma, a person cycles between crises and crisis behavior on the one pole and emotional suppression on the other.

TIP

A common reason that people experience unrelenting crises is that they have difficulty with *discernment* in relationships, meaning that some people seem to have a poorer capacity to assess whether another person is kind or self-interested. If this resonates for you, you are much more likely to be drawn into harmful relationships, and this is where you and your therapist can help identify the warning signs that predict an unhealthy relationship or situation.

Dialectical thinking is critical when working through all of these dilemmas. Your task is to recognize that you are stuck in one extreme of the polarities as a first step. Then see the ways in which your experiences may seem contradictory (for instance, "I know exactly what I need to do, but I just can't do it," or "I am an emotionally sensitive person, but I tell myself I shouldn't be," and so on).

The first step is developing a mindset allows you to recognize the coexistence of these polarities — see Worksheet 11-1.

Worksheet 11-1   My Experience of the Dialectical Dilemmas

PRACTICE

Review the dialectical dilemmas just covered. Write down the dilemmas that you identify with. Then identify the behaviors that occur in each polarity.

My emotional vulnerability:

_____

_____

The ways in which I self-invalidate:

_____

_____

The ways in which I am actively passive and let things get so bad that others do the things I need to do:

_____

_____

The ways in which I am apparently competent as manifest by being able to express myself and explain what I need, but I can't actually do the things I need to:

_____

_____

The ways in which crisis behavior manifests in my life:

_____

_____

The sorrows, traumas, and losses that I have avoided or not have yet to deal with:

_____

_____

Working Through Your Dialectical Dilemmas

Now that you have identified which of these dilemmas apply to you, what comes next? DBT offers a comprehensive toolbox of skills and strategies that can help you deal with your dialectical dilemmas, and by the time you've reached this chapter, many of these ideas should be familiar. You've learned the skills and now you need to practice them; otherwise, you'll end up falling into *apparent competence*, a dilemma that you just learned about!

Dealing with emotional vulnerability

REMEMBER

Emotional vulnerability is mostly about your biology and typically manifests as an extreme sensitivity to emotional stimuli, such as having strong, enduring, and painful emotional reactions to seemingly small events. It can include difficulty in controlling any behavior that is associated with the underlying emotions, such as your facial expressions or verbal and physical lashing out. See Worksheet 11-2.

PRACTICE

Worksheet 11-2   My Physical Reactions to Emotions

As with many practices in this book, the first step involves noticing, and mindfulness is the best skill to help you notice. Noticing is the associated mindfulness practice of participating fully by accepting that you are as you are, and your emotions are a part of you. Write down the ways in which you are sensitive, and, ideally, write down the ways that your body reacts to emotions.

_____

_____

_____

_____

_____

_____

_____

TIP

It is very important that you pay attention to the ways that certain vulnerability factors impact your biology. Highly sensitive people tend to have much bigger reactions to poor sleep, hunger, drugs, alcohol, and lack of exercise. See Worksheet 11-3.

PRACTICE

Worksheet 11-3   How my Emotions Are Impacted by Sleep Quality

Write down the ways your emotions and your emotional expressions are impacted by your sleep quality, eating, drug use, and so on.

_____

_____

_____

_____

_____

_____

_____

Dealing with self-invalidation

REMEMBER

Self-invalidation involves rejecting, dismissing, or discounting your emotional experiences. You might also feel that you "should" be able to solve your problems easily, just because everyone else can, and in this context self-invalidation can include the behavior of looking to others to see how you "should" be acting or feeling. See Worksheet 11-4.

WARNING

Once you identify the pattern, you might initially find it difficult to change your self-invalidating behavior. Don't judge yourself. You have likely been self-invalidating for a long time. Stay with the practice of simply pointing it out. This is the key to overcoming self-invalidation.

Worksheet 11-4 My Negative Self-Talk and Negative Self-Judgments

PRACTICE Notice any negative self-talk and judgments. This is one of the many areas where the practice of mindfulness will help you. Write down all the ways in which you say, "I should not feel. . . ., I should be able to. . . .," or judge yourself for feeling or behaving a certain way.

_____

_____

_____

_____

_____

_____

_____

_____

_____

_____

_____

_____

_____

_____

The next step is to replace the self-invalidating language. For example, if you notice that you say things like "I shouldn't be so upset about . . ." notice that you *are* upset, and then you need to identify all the ways in which it actually makes sense that you are feeling this way. See Worksheet 11-5.

PRACTICE

Worksheet 11-5   Replacing Judgments with Observable Facts

Write down all the biological, temperamental, relational, and environmental factors that have led you to feel the way you do. For instance, if you are an emotionally sensitive person who has experienced rejections, and you are struggling with a big project at work and haven't been sleeping well, and then your friend cancels a dinner date, it would make sense that you feel upset *even if* others think that you are making a big deal of the situation.

What are ways that you can replace "I shouldn't or should . . ." with "it makes sense that I do feel this way given the following factors. . ."

_____

_____

_____

_____

_____

_____

_____

_____

_____

_____

Dealing with active passivity

REMEMBER

In effect, active passivity is when you stop trying to solve a problem or use maladaptive approaches to solve a problem and instead wait for the problem to get bad enough that others step in to solve the problem for you. Others end up fixing the problem because they are worried about the consequences. See Worksheet 11-6.

Worksheet 11-6   The Task at Hand

Think about something that needs to get done where active passivity has shown up. Clarify your values around this issue and do this by asking yourself the following questions.

What are my emotional needs? Write down the emotions that get in the way of solving your problems and what you need in order to solve the problem of emotional excess.

_____

_____

_____

What are my personal responsibilities? Write down the elements of the situation that are your responsibility to solve.

_____

_____

_____

What is essential for my own personal self-care? What are the self-care actions that I need to take in order to feel that I am at my best? Sleep? Eating? Exercise?

_____

_____

_____

Once you have completed the previous practice, try these tips:

>> **Make lists:** Write down the thing that you have to get done and what you need to get the thing done. For instance, if you have to apply for a job, you need to complete an application and have an up-to-date resume.

>> **Be realistic:** What are all the things going on in your life right now? Is it essential to focus on all of them at this moment? Are there things that you can delay until after you have completed the task that needs to get done? Write down all the obligations in your life and prioritize the critical ones. Then focus on the task and be realistic as to what can actually be

done in the time that you have. Reprioritize less time-sensitive obligations until you have completed what you need to do.

>> **Take baby steps:** Often, when you have delayed or avoided the task at hand, it can seem a lot bigger than it once seemed. Break the task down into smaller steps. For instance, if you are applying for a job and it includes a four-page application, start by completing the first page and then give yourself a break before tackling the next page.

TIP

If you feel that you are out of control when problems arise, you're likely to end up on the active passivity pole of the dilemma. This is because when problems come up and you're emotionally dysregulated, you're more likely to feel at a loss as to what to do, and then wait for someone else to address the problem.

REMEMBER

Being actively passive can lead to more stress in the long run. This is because letting problems fester without dealing with them will typically cause them to grow, which will, in turn, cause you to feel more overwhelmed and less in control, which doesn't actually teach you how to solve problems. Know that if you leave it to the last moment, have a crisis, and then have someone else completes the application for you, you are simply reinforcing active passivity. Active passivity also paves the path toward shame, which then makes a person more vulnerable to swinging to the other side.

Dealing with apparent competence

Remember that apparent competence refers to a person's tendency to appear capable and skilled. They are able to "talk-the-talk" by saying the things that show insight, and that they know what to do. However, they struggle to put this apparent knowledge and competence into action. Use Worksheet 11-7 to identify all your competencies — apparent, real, and contextual.

PRACTICE

Worksheet 11-7   My True Competencies

First of all, you have real competence: Write down all the things that you are capable of doing, things like art, writing, gardening, music, and so on. What are your real competencies?

_____

_____

_____

_____

_____

_____

Next, write down your contextual competencies. These are the things that you can do when you are feeling emotionally and interpersonally stable, but you find much more difficult when you are distressed — maybe activities like homework, housework, and social obligations. In these cases, your competence is context dependent. When do you exhibit contextual competence?

_____

_____

_____

_____

_____

_____

_____

Now focus on where you show apparent competence. For instance, you might know your DBT skills extremely well but are unable to use them when you need to, or you can explain exactly what you need to do to complete a college application, but when it comes to actually doing it you can't. These are examples of apparent competence. What are ways in which you know what to do but can't do it? These are situations that often confuse others because they are convinced that you are capable but can't understand why it's so difficult for you.

_____

_____

_____

_____

(continued)

_____

_____

_____

_____

_____

_____

Dealing with unrelenting crises

WARNING

Dealing with this pole of the dilemma can be very hard on your own. Typically it's best to work with a therapist to address this. Doing this on your own is like just having learned how to swim and then attempting to swim in a stormy ocean. Having a therapist who can help figure this out is like having a swim coach in the swimming analogy. Use Worksheet 11-8 to document your various crises.

Worksheet 11-8   My Crises Situations

PRACTICE

Your first step is to document your various crises. Unrelenting means that you move from one crisis to the next, with very little time to settle between each crisis. Write down some of the stressful and emotionally overwhelming situations that you have experienced in the past week or month.

_____

_____

_____

_____

_____

_____

_____

_____

The next step, once you have documented the crises, is to write down all that you can about the various situations — the people, the places, the time of day, your vulnerability factors, including sleep and hunger, if drugs were involved, if you used target behaviors, and so on. Be as clear as you can in describing each of these situations. (Remember that _target behaviors_ are the behaviors that you want to change because they are getting in the way of realizing your hopes and goals.)

_____

_____

_____

_____

_____

_____

_____

_____

(continued)

_____

_____

_____

_____

_____

Next, write down whether there are any common themes that show up with these crises: Are the same people involved? Do crises occur in the same place? Are drugs involved, and so on. Your goal is to identify any patterns.

_____

_____

_____

_____

_____

_____

_____

_____

Next, if you begin to see a pattern, ask yourself if are there concrete steps that you can take ahead of time to ensure that you don't slip into the same pattern. For example, if crisis situations happen whenever you are with a specific person, are there things that you can do to change that pattern? For instance, can you stop meeting with that person? Communicate directly using interpersonal effectiveness skills with that person? Change how often you see that person? If you have found a pattern to your crisis behaviors, write down the ways in which you can change some of the elements that contribute to the situation.

_____

_____

_____

_____

_____

_____

Finally, if you live in an extremely stressful environment — for example one where people are abusive and it would be difficult·to leave — can you discuss this with your therapist and see if you can come up with alternative ideas?

Dealing with inhibited grieving

The most effective way to get through the sorrow of loss or the pain of trauma is to fully experience the experience and emotions. You feel sad when you are sad, you ask for help when you need it, you engage in your life fully without avoiding painful emotions. However, for those who struggle with emotional suppression, the feelings and memories are so painful that it is not easy to do without help.

WARNING

When inhibited grieving is part of your experience, to the outside world, there is no indication that you are struggling. However, those emotions have to go somewhere. When you bury them deep inside, you are inhibiting the grieving process, and at some point, something will trigger the old memories or loss and your emotions will be overwhelming, putting you at risk for destructive behavior.

TIP

When the expression of grief is inhibited, it affects your psychological health as well as your physical health. It may manifest as physical symptoms, including headaches, stomach aches, digestive problems, muscle tension, feeling depleted or exhausted, difficulty sleeping, and other symptoms. Use Worksheet 11-9 to document your significant losses.

PRACTICE

Worksheet 11-9   Losses I Have Experienced

If you have experienced a significant loss, whether by death or because of the end of a relationship, start by acknowledging the loss. It is a painful task to do, and you can validate your pain. The first step in overcoming the inhibited grieving is to acknowledge that you have lost someone important to you. Write down the name of the person who is no longer in your life.

_____

Loss can also include the loss of a job, moving from your childhood home, moving on from college, and so on. If this is your loss, write it down.

My loss is ..._____

Of course, many people have more than one loss. Your task in this exercise is to focus on the losses that you are avoiding processing.

_____

_____

_____

_____

Next, your task is to fully experience the emotions that come with the loss, often a deep sadness and sorrow. Write down all the emotions that come up for you as you think about your loss.

_____

_____

_____

_____

_____

_____

TIP

If doing this exercise causes you more emotional pain than you think you can bear, do you have any ideas about what might help? Is there someone you could call who could sit with you? Is there an outdoor space that is soothing for you where you might feel better?

Use Worksheet 11-10 to express your gratitude for people who are no longer in your life.

Worksheet 11-10   Gratitude for the People No Longer in My Life

PRACTICE

Processing grief can include honoring the people who were meaningful in your life. You can also express gratitude for the ways they helped you grow as a person, the positive ways they shaped you. It makes sense that you would feel powerful emotions because of your loss. Write down all the ways in which you have gratitude for the person who is no longer in your life. This practice can be used for any loss, such as your health, the loss of community, the loss of a job, and so on.

_____

_____

_____

_____

_____

_____

_____

TIP

Remind yourself that grief and sorrow is a natural part of life. Remember that you would not feel the way you do had you not cared the way you did.

WARNING

If instead of loss of a relationship, the inhibited grief is secondary to significant trauma, it is very likely that you will need dedicated therapy for that trauma. Trauma therapy is beyond the scope of this workbook; however, the various trauma therapies are compatible with DBT, including prolonged exposure (PE), cognitive processing therapy (CPT), trauma focused cognitive behavior therapy (TF-CBT), eye movement desensitization and processing therapy (EMDR), and others.

Embracing the Paradox

A *paradox* is defined as a proposition or an idea that seems contradictory or even absurd at first glance but that on further examination or reflection, contains a possible truth. Psychology is full of paradoxes. From a DBT perspective, if you can connect with these without becoming stressed or confused by them, it can be a way to see the world in less polarized, all-or-nothing, black-and-white ways.

Similarly, dialectical dilemmas can be paradoxical in that they contain seemingly opposing views. Paradoxes are different from dialectical dilemmas (where the focus is on moments of struggles) in that by embracing paradoxes, you are developing a level of cognitive flexibility that illuminates a path to a life of completeness. Here are some examples:

» If you are a goal-driven person, you might want to become better at paying attention by spending months at a meditation retreat, only to end up disengaging with the rest of your life. The paradoxical resolution is that you neither have to go to a meditation retreat or disengage from the rest of your life, but rather see that the present moment is one that you can focus on. By practicing small moments of paying attention in your daily life, you can improve your attention.

» Maybe you realize that you get so much joy from the people, things, and experiences in your life, and you want more. The paradox is that joy is only experienced in your mind. It is not experienced outside of you, even if the event that brings you joy is outside of you. When you embrace the idea that the people, the things, and the experiences you have are representations and interpretations you have in your mind, you begin to see that you can start to conjure up pleasant memories of experiences and people, and that this too will elicit joy, even if you are not there or with the people. If you focus mainly on negative thoughts, try switching your focus of attention to positive experiences and memories. Over time, you will see that you can control your emotional experience this way.

» You recognize that in life there are so many things that you can't control, and yet you spend so much time trying to control outcomes. Think about it — you did not control your birth, you can't control your aging. You can't control what your boss will say to you tomorrow, whether there will be traffic on the way to work, and so on.

However, you have an opportunity to be fully present and engaged. You can control how you breathe; you can control how you attend to the next step you take; you can control the way you attend to drinking your tea or coffee in the morning. The paradox is that rather than focusing on all the big things that you cannot change, focus on controlling the few things that you can. When you work on the small things, you will begin to see that your experience of the big things changes.

» You experience life as a separate person, independent of everything around you, and yet how could you exist without the air and the water or the food that you eat? What about the people who grow the food, who harvest it, who place it in trucks to take to market? The people who work in the markets and the stores, the bus driver who takes you to and from work, the people who built the bus, and the ones who built the roads. Think about yourself as just a tiny cog in a much bigger picture, because you are! Just like everybody else. Without your work you would not earn money that you spend on food and bus tickets and taxes, which keeps stores open, bus drivers employed, and roads built. We are all interdependent and a part of a much bigger picture. By embracing this paradox, you see your worth.

>> If you have children, you are a mother and a daughter, a father and a son. You are a link in a series of connections that go back to the beginning of time and might continue to the end of time. When you are with your mother, you act, feel, and think differently than when you are with your child, and yet you are the same person. When you embrace this paradox, you are free to be as you are under the conditions you are in.

After reflecting on these examples, consider your own experience, and see if any of them resonate. Use Worksheet 11-11 to help. Worksheet 11-12 can help you embrace your paradoxes.

PRACTICE

Worksheet 11-11   Paradoxes in My Life

Take a few ideas that you hold as firm truths, and ask yourself if you can see them in any other way. Practice flexibility in your thinking as a way to reduce any rigidity that causes you to suffer.

Don't start with the hardest paradoxes. Start with some easier ideas and then move to the harder ones. For example, how might you embrace the paradox of needing to exercise, knowing that you will feel more energized and content when you do, and yet exhausted and without energy? Write down some examples and then try to see a different side to your initial point of view.

_____

_____

_____

_____

_____

_____

_____

_____

_____

(continued)

Worksheet 11-11 *(continued)*

_____

_____

_____

_____

_____

_____

_____

_____

_____

Your next task is to see if there is a way to reconcile the paradox in a healthy, value-driven, and goal-focused way. Let's continue with the previous example. You are exhausted and all you want to do is climb into bed and sleep. And yet you haven't exercised, and you know that you will feel less exhausted when you exercise. Yet again, the exercise that will energize you will also exhaust you! A paradox for sure. You see both sides of the paradox and you freeze without action. Let's consider the following options:

» You had an exhausting day at work, and your boss asked you to work overtime. You know that you have to get up early the next day. You know that exercise is important to you and that you feel better when you do it. Perhaps you can take a day off — your body is telling you that it needs to rest!

Alternatively, if you feel that you must exercise, can you change it up? Rather than running three miles, run two. Rather than an hour in the gym, do half an hour.

» You're binge watching your favorite show and you're feeling lazy. It's a pleasant day out, and you know that going to the gym, going for a brisk walk or jog, will help you feel better. Can you use willingness and opposite action to get up and do your workout?

Alternatively, can you set a limit to watch a certain number of episodes and commit to shutting off your screen and exercising after that?

Better yet, can you turn off your screen right now, finish your exercise routine, and then reward yourself with a few episodes of your show?

» If you are bored of your exercise routine, can you think about mixing it up? If you walk, can you swim? If you do yoga, can you take a few classes in kickboxing?

» If you struggle with commitment to exercise, can you connect with a person who also wants to exercise and agree that you will support each other?

PRACTICE

Worksheet 11-12   Ways to Embrace My Paradoxes

Now that you have an idea of how to embrace a paradoxical situation, use one of your examples from the previous exercise and consider various ways to tackle your conundrum. Remember that it is key to use *and* rather than *but* when proposing solutions. For instance: This is my circumstance AND I can do X, Y, or Z.

_____

_____

_____

_____

_____

_____

_____

_____

_____

_____

_____

4

It Doesn't End Here: Living a DBT Lifestyle

Chapter **12**

Living a Life without Mood-Dependent Behaviors

For many people who come to DBT, mood-dependent behaviors are one of the symptoms that can wreak the most havoc. Mood-dependent behaviors occur when your mood, instead of your goals and values, dictates your behaviors. You may find that when your mood is "good," you can go to work or school, engage with the people in your life, get to places when you say you will, complete tasks, meet deadlines, and follow through on your long- and short-term goals.

However, when your mood is low, when you are sad, anxious, angry, or feel feelings like shame and guilt, the people, commitments, and goals that were once important to you no longer feel that way. What is even harder is that not only do you not *feel* important, but you engage in behaviors that may demonstrate they are no longer important. Many people who struggle with mood-dependent behaviors often feel they are (and are told by others that they are) unreliable, inconsistent, and only care about their own needs and wants. These are very painful things to hear.

Using DBT Skills to Regulate Your Emotions

As briefly discussed in Chapter 6, mood-dependent behaviors stem from the *emotion mind*, which is when you look at the world only through the lens of how you feel right now and what you need in that very moment. You quickly let go of anything that does not provide more immediate relief. Learning and practicing the DBT skills of mindfulness, emotion regulation, distress tolerance, and interpersonal effectiveness helps you learn to understand and regulate your emotions and urges. That way, mood-dependent behavior becomes a choice you may make from time to time, not something you feel compelled to do. DBT helps you find freedom from a life where your emotions dictate too many of your behaviors!

In addition to your DBT skills, there are other tools that this chapter explains to help you live more effectively. These skills will increase your confidence and ability to live a life with fewer mood-dependent behaviors:

>> Learning to set wise-minded goals

>> Breaking down large tasks and goals into steps

>> Managing your motivation

>> Thinking about and planning for obstacles

Wisely Setting Goals

Setting goals is not always easy, and often it is more complicated than it seems. Setting a goal that requires you to change your behavior often requires that you give up an old behavior and learn a new one. People forget that even if the behavior is ineffective or they are not doing something they "should be doing," there is still a reason they are doing it.

In Chapter 5, you learned all about functions of behavior and reinforcement. Those principles will help you set goals and understand why you are not changing behaviors despite many reasons that you should. As you set your goals, remember to look for the function of your old behavior and validate the challenges of the changes that lie ahead. Sometimes, problem behaviors are providing solutions to something else!

When setting goals (see Worksheet 12-1), ask yourself the following questions:

>> What is my goal?

>> What do I want to accomplish by setting this goal?

>> Why do I want to work on this goal now?

>> What are the pros and cons to setting this goal or keeping things as is (you can review pros and cons in Chapter 9)?

>> Do I need to set an intermediate goal?

>> What emotions am I noticing and can I validate?

Worksheet 12-1   Setting a Wise Goal

Use this worksheet to follow the goal-setting questions and set a goal you would like to work on in the next week.

1.   What is my goal?

_____

_____

_____

_____

2.   What do I want to accomplish by setting this goal?

_____

_____

_____

_____

3.   Why do I want to work on this goal now?

_____

_____

_____

_____

(continued)

Worksheet 12-1 *(continued)*

4. What are the pros and cons to setting this goal or keeping things as is?

Pros	Cons

5. Do I need to set an intermediate goal? If so, what is it?

_____

_____

_____

_____

6. What emotions am I noticing that I can validate?

_____

_____

_____

_____

Breaking Down the Steps

One of the things that can trip people up when setting goals is that completing the goal seems overwhelming. Once you set a wise-minded goal, you need to step back and consider the steps that you must take to get there.

The first thing you want to consider is a realistic timeline. How long do you think this will take or when would you like to complete the goal? Once you have a timeline, identify the tasks or smaller steps that you need to complete. Next, prioritize the tasks and ensure they are in an practical order to help you move toward completing your goal. Place each task on the timeline so that you can identify deadlines. Next, you need recognize when you accomplish each of these steps. You have learned that positive reinforcement can help you continue to be effective. Continue to work through each step until you complete your goal (see Worksheet 12-2).

REMEMBER

Remember to be open to feedback and suggestions along the way.

Worksheet 12-2   Taking My Goal from an Idea to Action

Use this worksheet to practice breaking down your goal into steps and using a timeline to make a plan.

1. What is your timeline? Remember to be mindful of a realistic amount of time to reach your goal. Think about what is going on in your life, the lives of people you need to help you, and the availability of any resources you may need.

    _____

    _____

    _____

    _____

2. Break down your goal into smaller steps. What are those steps?

    _____

    _____

    _____

(continued)

_____

_____

3. Add your steps and tasks to your timeline. Prioritize the tasks accordingly and indicate when you will complete each step.

_____

_____

_____

_____

4. What are your reinforcers? How will you reward yourself or celebrate when you complete a step that brings you closer to your goal?

_____

_____

_____

_____

Maintaining Motivation

There are many factors that impact your motivation. Some of the most common things influencing your motivation are your mood or psychological state, the environment that you are in, and your history of achievement and perseverance. In DBT and in life, motivation helps you persevere when things get challenging so that you can continue to reach your goals. When you maintain motivation, it helps you increase your self-confidence, helps you continue to strive to achieve your goals, gives you a sense of purpose, helps you overcome challenges, and encourages you to be more skillful in general. Setting wise goals will help you stay motivated!

WARNING

There are several factors that lead to loss of motivation — the biggest one often being your mood, which is why many people with mood-dependent behaviors struggle with motivation. It is important to be mindful of how your mood is connected to your motivation. There may be some mood states that differentially impact your motivation. Pay attention to your own red flags that indicate your motivation is waning. Some common red flags of mood-dependent behaviors are feelings of disappointment when things do not go as you had hoped or expected, anger, sadness/depression, fear of being rejected or judged, fear of failure, and disgust and self-loathing.

If you notice your motivation failing, consider the *building mastery* skill from emotion regulation (see Chapter 7). Building mastery is a way to increase your self-confidence because you are doing something that is challenging and makes you feel accomplished. If your mood is low, consider the *opposite action* skill as well, which is covered in Chapter 7. Opposite action helps you when your mood is getting in the way of being effective and moving toward your goals (see Worksheets 12-3 and 12-4).

Here are some ideas to consider when you are losing motivation:

>> Consider skills like building mastery and opposite action.

>> Keep your mind on your long-term goal and remind yourself why it is important to you in your wise mind.

>> Remember your effective and successful behaviors in the past. Look at the smaller steps you have accomplished!

>> Be kind to yourself and self-validate.

Worksheet 12-3   Signs I Am Losing Motivation

Use this worksheet to identify the emotions, thoughts, and behaviors that are signs that you are losing motivation. Remember, being aware of your red flags will help you use adaptive skills sooner, which will make regaining motivation easier.

Red Flags: Emotions	Red Flags: Thoughts	Red Flags: Behaviors

Worksheet 12-4   My Skills Plan for Warning Signs and Loss of Motivation

Now that you have identified your red flags that lead to loss of motivation, use this worksheet to identify skills to address them. Transcribe your red flags from Worksheet 12-3 and use this chapter as well as Chapters 5-9 to identify skills from the DBT modules. This is a great way to practice applying these skills!

My Red Flags: Emotions:

_____

_____

Skills I Can Use:

_____

_____

_____

My Red Flags: Thoughts:

_____

_____

_____

Skills I Can Use:

_____

_____

_____

My Red Flags: Behaviors:

_____

_____

_____

Skills I Can Use:

_____

_____

_____

Observing Obstacles

While being aware of and observing obstacles can be hard, doing so can help you avoid mood-dependent behaviors when something gets in the way of your plan. When you hit an obstacle, you may notice a surge in emotions that makes you want to change your plan or even give up. Most people have certain emotions and thought patterns that show up when they hit an obstacle.

Some people notice thoughts of being a failure, nothing goes my way, things are too hard, or I'm not meant to be successful. These are the kind of thoughts that can make your motivation nose-dive. Sometimes you can anticipate obstacles and sometimes you cannot. Powerful obstacles that can lead to mood-dependent behaviors are disappointment, shame, guilt, feeling left out, feeling regretful, or for many social media and plans changing. It is important to be mindful of obstacles you can anticipate (see Worksheet 12-5).

EXAMPLE

Natasha finds that when plans are changed at the last minute, she is at risk of mood-dependent behaviors. As a generally anxious person, Natasha thinks it's critical to know her plans for the day so that she can cope ahead and be prepared. When the plans change, like friends change restaurants or decide to add on another activity, her anxiety rises and she gets angry, stops responding to texts, and often doesn't show up. It is for this reason that her friends don't always invite her and that she has developed a bit of a reputation for being unreliable. She is often lonely and doesn't like that her friends think she is "high maintenance." Since learning DBT, Natasha is working on staying present and using coping ahead and opposite action to keep her plans, even when there are changes that make her anxious. She wants to be a more reliable friend.

Worksheet 12-5   My Reflections on Obstacles

Use this worksheet to write about the kinds of obstacles that you find challenging, how you have responded, and how you would like to respond more skillfully.

_____

_____

_____

_____

_____

_____

_____

_____

_____

_____

_____

_____

Eliminating Emotional Decision Making

Emotional decision making is a mood-dependent behavior that stems from the emotion mind, covered in Chapter 6. Emotional decision making is a tell-tale sign of mood-dependent behavior, as you are making decisions based on how you feel in the moment and not considering your longer-term goals, relationships, pros and cons, or what you know to be true in your wise mind. Emotional decision making can lead to short- and long-term negative consequences that — once you return to a wise mind — you may have to manage.

Eliminating emotional decision making starts with the mindful awareness using *observe* and *describe* that you learned in Chapter 6. Emotions will arise in the face of your decision making — the question is, can you step back and assess if they are emotions that will help you make wise decisions or emotions that will get in the way and lead you to emotional decision making? The good news is that if you can catch the emotions that will send you astray, you can notice them and use your skills to find your wise mind.

TIP

One of the biggest pieces of advice we can give you about this is that strong emotions make you want to move quickly, so to avoid emotional decision making, you must *SLOW DOWN!*

Consider the following tips to avoid emotional decision making:

>> Be aware of when you are in your emotion mind. What are your emotion mind red flags? Look back at your work in Chapter 6.

>> Practice noticing emotion mind urges to change a plan or a goal. Ask yourself, are these emotion minded solutions to this situation?

>> Self-validate the emotion that you are experiencing. What makes sense about the way you feel right now?

>> Slow down and take five deep breaths.

>> Remind yourself that you do not have to decide in this moment; you must first get regulated.

>> Find your wise mind. Sit somewhere quiet and ask your wise mind what the answer is.

>> Be mindful of what time it is! As the day goes on, your brain, along with the rest of your body, gets tired, which makes nighttime a high risk for emotion-minded decision making! See Worksheet 12-6.

Worksheet 12-6　Learning from Past Emotional Decisions

Use this worksheet to consider two times that you engaged in emotional decision making recently. Using some of the previous tips — what could you have done to notice and shift your emotion mind? What about the decision would have been different, and what would have been the same?

Past Emotional Decision #1:

_____

_____

_____

_____

Ways I could have been mindful of my emotion mind before making a decision:

_____

_____

_____

Would practicing these skills have made an impact on my decision? If yes, how so? If no, why not?

_____

_____

_____

Past Emotional Decision #2:

_____

_____

_____

_____

Ways I could have been mindful of my emotion mind before making a decision:

_____

_____

_____

_____

Would practicing these skills have made an impact on my decision? If yes, how so? If no, why not?

_____

_____

_____

_____

Chapter **13**

Focusing on Future Self

Throughout this book, you have learned skills with the goal of being a more effective self. This chapter turns things around so you can look back at yourself from the future; a future where you are more effective and managing all of life's challenges with skill and self-respect.

Identifying the Person You Want to Be

Consider the person you want to be as your *future self*. Your future self is the version of you who exists in the future beyond the present moment. It is the *you* that you want to be in the coming days, weeks, months, and years.

Your future self is a concept that involves imagining the person you want to be. This includes considering your future achievements, self-respect, effective and adaptive behaviors, as well as healthy and mutually beneficial relationships.

REMEMBER

The goal in picturing a future you is to focus on and behave in ways that align with your values and long-term goals. In so doing, you create a bridge between the *you* you are now and the *you* you want to be.

There is research on the concept of future self, and, if you think about it, there are multiple alternative versions of who you might turn out to be. Imagine that you are driving on the interstate on a cross-country trip. You come to a big intersection, and you can go North, South, East, or West. The choice you make will mean that you will have different experiences, meet different people, taste different foods, stay at different hotels, encounter different landscapes, and so on.

You can never know exactly which path will work out better for you, only that the outcome of each path will be different. What is important, however, is to have some degree of clarity as to what your goals and intentions are. If you are driving from Boston to Los Angeles, with California being your goal, turning South and driving to Florida is not consistent with your goal. Or, perhaps, you want to make a detour, and that is okay, but the you who took the detour will be different from the one who didn't.

What is also interesting to consider is that your future self is shaped by your dreams, your fears, your opportunities, your fantasies, and your regrets, and knowing all this about yourself will give you a leg up in determining the vision of your future self.

Benefits of Connecting with Your Future Self

Connecting with your future self can serve as a landmark. By knowing where you want to go, you know the things that you need to know (and do) now. Imagine that you are unfit, but have the goal to hike to the top of a distant mountain. The top of the mountain is the landmark, the point that beckons you, and in this context, it tells you what you need to do now. You need to start exercising in this present moment. Imagine that the top of the mountain is a *you* that is effective and self-assured (see Worksheet 13-1). What are the steps that you need to take now to get to that point?

PRACTICE

Worksheet 13-1   My Future Me

Imagine you in the future, and remember, the future is any time from tomorrow to months or years from now. For the sake of this exercise, imagine the person you want to be. In the next few lines, write down the version of you that you want to be, that you imagine being proud of.

_____

_____

_____

_____

_____

_____

Connecting with your future self can spark your motivation. In addition to having the future you being a beacon — a landmark that you can see in the distance of time — it can also be your source of motivation. The thoughts of a future self can be the pull that motivates you to continue to practice DBT skills.

Connecting with your future self also helps you focus on wisdom. In DBT, the wise mind is a deep well of wisdom that guides decisions. It prompts you to integrate your emotions and rational minds, and in so doing, ensures that your present actions boost your chances of fulfilling your future goals.

Connecting with your future self also helps you underemphasize your short-term goals. By focusing on your future self, you are less likely to prioritize short-term rewards, or short-term behavioral benefits, especially if they are not consistent with your long-term goals. For instance, hooking up with multiple partners may feel good in the moment, but may be inconsistent with the development of a steady, healthy relationship (with yourself and others). Try Worksheet 13-2.

Worksheet 13-2   My Harmful Short-Term Behaviors

PRACTICE

Write down any behaviors that give you short-term benefit, but that are not consistent with your dreams or your future self. These behaviors could include target skills, such as substance use, dangerous sexual behaviors, overeating, self-injury, and so on.

_____

_____

_____

_____

_____

Connecting with your future self enhances your persistence. With enhanced persistence, you are better able to overcome challenges and endure what you need to do now, which will help you get to that future you. If you think about getting to the top of the mountain in the previous example, there will certainly be easy sections along the path, but there will also be steep and rocky sections, and these are the moments when you need to persist.

Connecting with your future self helps you make more effective choices. When you focus on your future self, you can ask yourself whether your present behavior will benefit you on your path. In the mountain analogy, there may be times when you need to slow down, stop to rest, or when you need to nourish your body. Consider the behaviors that you are doing now, and ask yourself whether they are beneficial and consistent with your goals. Try to identify any behaviors that are not consistent with your goals. See Worksheet 13-3.

Worksheet 13-3   Identifying My Current Behaviors

PRACTICE

Write down a list of common behaviors that you do on a regular basis, and then consider whether these behaviors are consistent with your vision of your future self.

_____

_____

_____

_____

_____

_____

_____

_____

Finally, connecting with your future self increases accountability. Imagine your future self speaking to you. Would that future version of you be proud of what you are doing right now? Can future you hold you accountable for your present actions? Can you turn your future self into a friend who supports you — someone who encourages you to make decisions that are in your best interest?

What about your former self?

Making sure that you don't slip back into harmful past-self behaviors is critical for your personal growth, for intentional decision making, and for knowing yourself.

REMEMBER Your former self is a representation of how your biological development interacted with your past experiences, behaviors, choices, and interactions. The only benefit to reflecting on your former self is to learn from the mistakes you made and the way in which you succeeded. However, your past self does not determine what your future will be. It is not a representation of who you will be become.

Even though your former self does not predict who your future self will be, your former self, former behaviors, and former relationships have brought you to your present self. *Mindful self-awareness* is the act of becoming aware of your current self — made up your beliefs, values, strengths, and weaknesses. Think about how often your former self paid careful attention to who you were. Many people who come to DBT do not believe that they have much to offer the world, but this is a faulty way of thinking and one to pay attention to. Everyone has something valuable they can share, and when you are aware, you can see it. Use Worksheet 13-4 to examine your true nature.

Worksheet 13-4   Considering My True Nature

PRACTICE Take ten minutes to examine your true nature. Write down your values, your current actions and reactions, the nature of your relationships, your strengths, and your weaknesses.

_____

_____

_____

_____

_____

_____

_____

_____

_____

_____

Avoiding the future self traps

TIP

There are some traps that you could fall into when you are considering your future self:

>> **Temporal discounting:** This is the tendency to place more value on near-term benefits and less value on future benefits, and it can lead you to prioritize short-term rewards over long-term ones. This is an excellent place to use the stop skill and then pros and cons to determine if temporal discounting is in play.

>> **Identity and continuity:** When you think about who you will be tomorrow, if you are like most people, you tend to view your tomorrow self as an extension of your current self. If you take this type of thinking into account, you will see that you are not simply an extension of your 2-, 5-, 10-, 15-year-old self. Yes, there are likely similarities, but there are many differences as well. If you spend your time worrying that your future self will be as unskilled as or suffer as much as your present self, you are less likely to be motivated to do the hard work now that your future self needs. Your identity does not automatically continue into the future. Don't let your brain trick you.

>> **Empathy for your present self:** If you don't have empathy or compassion for your present self, and you believe that your future self will simply be an older version of your present self, you might not be inclined to do something for a future you that you don't care about. However, if you can continue to work on believing that by being more skillful, you will suffer less, and that in so doing that future you will be grateful, that shows compassion and empathy for the more skilled future version of you. Stay compassionate for future you.

Use Worksheet 13-5 to visualize your future self.

THE PRINCIPLE OF IMPERMANENCE

One of the core principles of DBT is the *principle of impermanence*. Everything changes, and this present moment will change. Who you were in the past is not who you are now. Look back at pictures of yourself a year ago, five years ago, even ten years ago. You can see how you change over the years — not just your physical self, but your emotional and psychological self as well. Everything has changed and will continue to do so into the future. The more you practice a skillful way of being, the more skillful your future self will be.

Worksheet 13-5   Visualizing My Future Self

PRACTICE

Try to create a complete mental image of your future self. There are various ways to do this. You can write down a future you with all the characteristics that you want future you to have, ones that you can work on in your DBT work. If you are an artist, draw future you. You might want to create music that captures future you. Your imagination is a powerful tool, and you can use it to visualize and create a future you that captures the best of your values and virtues.

_____

_____

_____

_____

_____

TIP

Research shows that people who are motivated by healthy future goals and who have strong positive emotions are more likely to behave in ways that benefit their long-term emotional and physical well-being. Review the visualization you created in this exercise and consider which behaviors are consistent with attaining that future self. Write down your healthy behaviors — the ones that you imagine a future you would be proud of.

_____

_____

_____

_____

_____

_____

(continued)

By connecting your present actions to the outcomes you want, you can set both short- and long-term goals that are realistic. Make a map of your future goals and present behaviors and draw arrows between your present behaviors and those future goals to see if they truly connect. (Chapter 3 talks more about setting goals.)

_____

_____

_____

_____

Recognizing Present-Self Behaviors

Try this thought experiment. If you don't have a vision of your future self, and you spend no time imagining the person you want to be, two things happen:

» First, you spend a lot of time dwelling in present behaviors, ones that may be keeping you stuck in suffering.

» Second, you end up being a victim and might just end up adapting to whatever life throws at you.

In order to become the version you are aiming to be, you have to start to recognize your present-self behaviors. Every one of our actions is goal-driven. With the practice of mindful self-assessment, you can know what your goal is simply by paying attention to your intentions by observing your own behavior. Your behavior is always driven by a commitment to a goal.

However, what if these behaviors are risky to your physical or emotional health? This is where it gets tricky. How can these behaviors possibly have any benefit?

Defining risky behaviors

What is the difference between a value-driven and goal-driven behavior and a risky behavior? One big difference is that risky behaviors have the potential for negative consequences. What sets risky behaviors apart is that they are inherently potentially dangerous and the likelihood that a bad outcome or harm will occur is high. Risky behaviors lead to danger and the possibility of harm or adverse outcomes. Risky behaviors encompass a wide range of actions that have the potential for negative consequences.

Many people who come to DBT experience the following behaviors:

>> Risky and potentially dangerous sexual behaviors

>> Excessive and risky drug and alcohol use

>> Harmful eating behaviors like restricting, bingeing, and purging

>> Reckless spending of money

>> Dangerous driving

>> Self-injury

>> Suicidal ideation and behavior

How are these behaviors consistent with a commitment to a goal? Let's break some of these down. Then you complete the worksheet after each section.

TIP

In the following worksheets, when assessing the *why* or purpose of the behavior, your task is to examine the emotions or experiences that you want to change by doing the behaviors. This takes some mindful self-awareness. For some ideas about why you might engage in risky behaviors, see the section later in this chapter entitled "Why do people engage in risky behaviors?"

>> **Unsafe and dangerous sexual practices:** These behaviors increase the risk of developing sexually transmitted infections, which can in turn lead to secondary infections and inflammation. They can lead to unwanted pregnancy or infertility. They can also lead to coercion and non-consent of sexual behavior, rape and physical violence, and feelings of degradation, shame, or lack of self-worth. Use Worksheet 13-6 to identify your dangerous sexual behaviors.

Worksheet 13-6   My Dangerous Sexual Behaviors

PRACTICE

Do you engage in dangerous sexual behaviors? If so, write these down and then identify the ways in which they have impacted you in terms of physical and emotional health and your sense of self.

_____

_____

_____

_____

_____

(continued)

Worksheet 13-6 *(continued)*

Next, identify when these behaviors show up and consider their function — or *why* you engage in these behaviors. For some food for thought, see the section later in this chapter entitled, "Why do people engage in risky behaviors?"

_____

_____

_____

_____

_____

_____

>> **Harmful eating behaviors:** These behaviors can cause significant health problems if left unaddressed: Restrictive eating can lead to a full-blown eating disorder such as anorexia nervosa, which can heart problems, low blood pressure, low body temperature, low blood sugar, low bone density, depression, and death. Bulimia, is where a person binges food and then purges it. This can lead to severe heartburn, dental problems from chronic vomiting, and loss or depletion of certain essential minerals and vitamins. Low potassium levels can be life threatening. Many people also purge soon after taking their medication, which then means that the medication will not be absorbed, and they will have no medication, or an inadequate level of medication in their system.

And finally, there is bingeing or overeating. There are various consequences to overeating, some of which temporarily feel good. Bingeing on a favorite snack means that you focus on the deliciousness of the taste, without attention to the long-term impact of consuming excess calories, Overeating can also lead to a feeling of sedation, which happens when the brain slows down to focus on digestion. In the short-term, overeating and bingeing feel good, but in the long-term they come at great physical and psychological cost. Use Worksheet 13-7 to identify your harmful eating behaviors.

Worksheet 13-7   My Harmful Eating Behaviors

PRACTICE

Do you engage in harmful eating behaviors? If so, write these down and then identify the ways in which they have impacted you in terms of physical and emotional health.

_____

_____

_____

_____

_____

Next, identify when these behaviors show up and consider their function — or *why* you engage in these behaviors. For some food for thought, see the section later in this chapter entitled, "Why do people engage in risky behaviors?"

_____

_____

_____

_____

_____

_____

_____

>> **Dangerous driving:** This can take various forms, from speeding to distracted driving, to driving under the influence to disregarding traffic laws. These are all behaviors that increase the likelihood of you having an accident and injuring yourself or other people. Use Worksheet 13-8 to identify your dangerous driving behaviors.

PRACTICE

Worksheet 13-8   My Dangerous Driving Behaviors

Do you engage in dangerous driving? If so, write the ways in which you do and then identify the ways in which these behaviors have impacted you and others.

_____

_____

_____

_____

_____

Next, identify when these behaviors show up and consider their function — or *why* you engage in these behaviors. For some food for thought, see the section later in this chapter entitled, "Why do people engage in risky behaviors?"

_____

_____

_____

_____

_____

_____

>> **Spending money recklessly:** This is another risky behavior. It includes making impulsive purchases, taking on excessive debt, or failing to save any money for the future. When these things happen, it can lead to loss of credit-worthiness, emotional stress, and even financial ruin. Use Worksheet 13-9 to identify any reckless money-spending behaviors you have.

Worksheet 13-9   My Money-Spending Behaviors

Do you spend money in a reckless way? If so, write the ways in which you do and the impact it has on you, specifically your overall financial health, as well as your loved ones.

_____

_____

_____

_____

_____

Next, identify when these behaviors show up and consider their function — or *why* you engage in reckless spending. For some food for thought, see the section later in this chapter entitled, "Why do people engage in risky behaviors?"

_____

_____

_____

_____

_____

_____

>> **Alcohol and drug misuse:** There is a mountain of research on the impact of the misuse of alcohol and other substances. At a macro level, misuse of drugs and alcohol reduces a person's life expectancy by ten years.

WHAT EXACTLY IS MISUSE?

The concept of *misuse* is twofold. The first definition is use that is not contextually or culturally normative. For instance, say a person has a glass of wine with dinner. There is no misuse then. However, let's say that the person, rather than deal with an important issue, has a glass of wine. That would be considered misuse (because they are self-medicating). The second definition is impact or functional consequence. Say that two people have a glass of wine with dinner. One is totally fine after dinner, but the impact on the second person is that they become belligerent. That second person is misusing the wine.

However, most people don't consider the impact on life-expectancy, reasoning that if their life is one of suffering, why should they want to live any longer than they have to? You don't have to look to the end of your life to see how drugs and alcohol impact it. There are many psychological and physical consequences of misusing substances. There can be trauma, liver and stomach issues, addiction issues, fetal alcohol syndrome in babies of women who drink alcohol during pregnancy, as well as increased risk of anxiety, depression, and suicidality in people who misuse drugs and alcohol. See Worksheet 13-10.

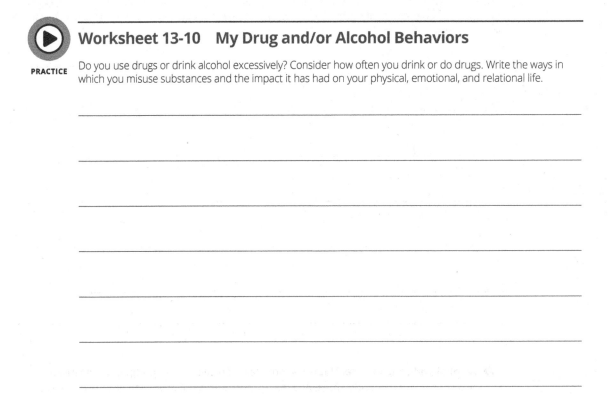

Worksheet 13-10   My Drug and/or Alcohol Behaviors

PRACTICE

Do you use drugs or drink alcohol excessively? Consider how often you drink or do drugs. Write the ways in which you misuse substances and the impact it has had on your physical, emotional, and relational life.

_____

_____

_____

_____

_____

_____

_____

Next, identify when these behaviors show up and consider their function — or *why* you engage in these behaviors. For some food for thought, see the section later in this chapter entitled, "Why do people engage in risky behaviors?"

_____

_____

_____

_____

_____

>> **Self-injury:** This is the deliberate/intentional destruction of body tissue. For people who come to DBT, the most common type of self-injury is cutting. This can lead to poor wound healing and infection, scarring, and, depending on where a person cuts, near-lethal, if not lethal, blood loss. Use Worksheet 13-11 to identify any self-injury behaviors you have.

▶ Worksheet 13-11   My Self-Injury Behaviors

PRACTICE

Do you self-injure? If so, how often do you do so, and where and how do you self-injure?

_____

_____

_____

_____

_____

(continued)

Worksheet 13-11 *(continued)*

Next, identify when these behaviors show up and consider their function — or *why* you engage in self-injury. For some food for thought, see the next section, entitled "Why do people engage in risky behaviors?"

_____

_____

_____

_____

_____

_____

Why do people engage in risky behaviors?

Now that you have reviewed your risky behaviors and considered the reasons you do them, this section covers what the research shows about the reasons for, or function of, these behaviors. There are various reasons people do risky behaviors.

Some people simply like the thrill of doing risky behaviors. It's one thing to do something risky for fun or for the kick of it, and another as a way of changing a psychological state of mind. It is important to distinguish between risky behaviors that don't require therapy and those that do. Some might say that parachute jumping, rock-climbing, extreme skiing, NASCAR racing, deep sea diving, going up in a hot-air balloon and many, many other behaviors are risky. There may be some risk to these behaviors, but under most circumstances, the people who engage in them are well trained and have a deep understanding of their craft.

These are not the types of behaviors we are talking about. If you are a talented downhill skier and feel safe on steep slopes, that is a competence and likely a behavior that brings you joy, and by all means you should continue. This section is about dangerous behaviors whereby you are typically not in control.

Typically, when this happens, it is for one of the following reasons:

>> **Fear of being alone or abandoned.** When this happens, you might engage in risky sexual behavior in order to feel connected and use sexual behaviors to keep another person close, even if temporarily.

>> **Wanting to feel connected.** For instance, you might agree to join a drinking game because your two best friends are drinking, and you feel that you will be less connected and feel judged by them if you don't drink, even if you know that drinking has serious consequences.

>> **Wanting to fit in at any cost.** You might be using substances in order to fit in with a social group, even if the substances don't bring pleasant feelings.

>> **Feeling numb.** Some people use pain in order to feel any kind of feeling rather the experience of feeling numb, which some describe as feeling dead.

>> **Feeling excessive and painful emotion.** The most common reason for self-injury is to calm excessive and painful emotions because self-injury has the effect of calming the brain. This can have a powerful, albeit very temporary calming effect.

>> **Not wanting to feel any emotions at all**. For instance, you might take an excessive amount of sedatives in order to feel numb or nothing at all, even at the risk of overdosing.

>> **Wanting to feel happier.** Some people will use substances, shopping, and dangerous driving in order to have their brain release its dopamine (feel-good chemical) stores.

>> **Wanting to feel control of something when you feel that you have no control at all.** This typically happens with eating disorders when a person feels that they have no control at all. They feel that they at least have control over how much they eat.

>> **Wanting to be seen.** On occasion, doing something risky or outrageous is a way to be seen. This can be a powerful reason when a person does not feel seen.

>> **Wanting others to know how bad you feel.** At times, although this is not a common reason, people will self-injure or attempt suicide in order to communicate to others just how much they are struggling.

If you want to change your behavior, you must start by acknowledging that you are doing it, and be honest with yourself about the consequences.

WARNING Engaging in risky and potentially dangerous behavior may provide temporary relief, excitement, and even pleasure, but if you don't pay attention to the longer-term emotional or physical consequences, you can experience physical injuries, infections, health complications, addictions, legal troubles, damaged or destroyed relationships, and even death. Use Worksheet 13-12 to contemplate your reasons for engaging in risky behavior.

Worksheet 13-12 My Reasons for Engaging in Risky Behavior

PRACTICE

After reading the reasons why people engage in risky behavior, review the behaviors you wrote about in the previous section and see if any of the functions/reasons listed apply to you and how.

_____

_____

_____

_____

_____

_____

_____

_____

_____

_____

Aligning Your Present and Future Self

You have reviewed the concept of your future self and your present-self behaviors. How do you align your present self with your future self? How do you ensure that you keep the behaviors that are helpful and reduce and change the behaviors that are not?

Start with your identity narrative. Your personality is the combination of your regular and consistent behavior, your beliefs, your reactions, and your emotions. When you think about your personality or identity, one way to consider it is to see it as a force that shapes you. Your _identity narrative_ is the way that you tell the story of you. The story of you includes your history, your interpretations, your current behaviors, and your interpretation of events. See Worksheet 13-13.

Reread your story. If you anchor who you are only in this story, the story of your past and present identity, you are creating a narrative and mindset that can feel permanent. By removing the anchor of stuckness and shifting your focus to the vision of your future self, you can begin to see the possibility of who you might be and create a beacon that can guide you there.

Worksheet 13-13   My Identity Narrative

What is the story of you? If someone were to ask you about yourself, what story would you tell them about the way you grew up, the things that happened to you, how you see yourself, the emotions you have, and the behaviors you do? Write this story down.

_____

_____

_____

_____

_____

_____

_____

_____

_____

_____

_____

_____

_____

_____

TIP

As you begin to align the *you* who you are today with the *you* that you will be in the future, be careful that you don't go too far out. For instance, if you are 25 years old, thinking about who you will be at 50 is too far away. The issue is that future you in the far, far away can seem too alien to be helpful. Make sure that you focus on a nearer-term future you, for instance, five years from now. Alternatively, you could focus on a year from now. DBT therapy usually lasts about a year, so if five years seems too far out, try one year.

Start by using Worksheet 13-14 to contemplate the qualities of other people that you admire.

PRACTICE

Worksheet 13-14   Accepting Admirable Qualities

If it feels overwhelming to imagine a very different and more skillful you, think of future you in the way that you might think of a close friend or someone you admire. Think about the qualities of that person you admire. Write down the qualities that you share and then consider whether you can develop the qualities that they have that you don't.

_____

_____

_____

_____

_____

_____

The next practice is to consider the qualities you have that you also admire in other people. For instance, say that you are a compassionate person, have a good sense of humor, and are a good listener. Consider that you want future you to continue to have those qualities. If the future you had the same level of compassion, sense of humor, and listening ability, would that be enough? If yes, all you need to do is continue doing what you are doing. If no, are there things you could do to be more compassionate? For instance, could you volunteer at a nonprofit? If you feel that you would want to improve your sense of humor, could you join an improv group or go to comedy clubs? If you want to be a better listener, can you consider the factors that are getting in the way of listening? For instance, do you tend to be in conversation with others with your phone in your hand?

Use Worksheet 13-15 to consider the qualities that you don't have in the present, but that you would like future you to have.

Worksheet 13-15   My Future Qualities and Abilities

PRACTICE

List the qualities or abilities you don't have now that you want future you to have and that you are committed to work toward.

_____

_____

_____

_____

_____

_____

_____

_____

Typically, for people who come to DBT, the qualities they would like their future selves to have include the following:

>> The ability to regulate emptions.

>> The ability to tolerate stressful moments.

>> The ability to maintain relationships.

>> The ability to feel confident with decisions.

>> The ability to have established values and live a value-driven life.

Use Worksheet 13-16 to identify the qualities you want to develop.

PRACTICE

Worksheet 13-16   Qualities I Need to Develop

Fill in the following table by identifying the qualities you want to develop and envisioning how your future you will use these qualities in stressful situations.

Qualities to Develop	Present You: Describe and Rank Your Present Ability on a Scale from 1-10	Future You: Describe How You Want Your Future Self to Act in Stressful Situations
Example: The ability to slow down before acting on an urge.	"I tend to be impulsive and not think." My ability to resist an urge is 2/10.	"My future self will be able to slow down and rapidly, confidently, and skillfully assess whether to act on urges or not."
Quality to develop # 1		
Quality to develop # 2		
Quality to develop # 3		

Qualities to Develop	Present You: Describe and Rank Your Present Ability on a Scale from 1-10	Future You: Describe How You Want Your Future Self to Act in Stressful Situations
Quality to develop # 4		
Quality to develop # 5		

Use Worksheet 13-17 to determine which DBT skills will help you get to your ideal future self.

Review the column of your present-self qualities and then write down all the skills and steps that you need to practice and focus on in order to progress, step-by-step, and day-by-day, to reach your future self. Then picture future you looking back at you today, thanking you!

PRACTICE

Worksheet 13-17   DBT Skills for Reaching My Future Self

Now that you have identified and described where you currently are and have a sense of the qualities you want future you to have, the final exercise in this chapter is to consider which DBT skills will help you get there.

For each of the qualities that you want to modify, consider the DBT skills that you will need to practice in order to become a more skillful future you. As an example, we filled in the grid with resisting the need to act on an urge. You might then determine that you need to develop your stop skill and practice the pros and cons of acting on a behavior, versus not acting on a behavior.

Quality to Develop	DBT Skills to Employ
Example: The ability to slow down before acting on an urge.	Develop the STOP skill and use Pros and Cons to determine how acting on this behavior will affect outcomes.
Quality to develop # 1	
Quality to develop # 2	

(continued)

Worksheet 13-17 *(continued)*

Quality to Develop	DBT Skills to Employ
Quality to develop # 3	
Quality to develop # 4	
Quality to develop # 5	

5

The Part of Tens

IN THIS PART . . .

Integrating DBT into your life beyond therapy and maintaining the gains you made

Overcoming obstacles like a pro

Practicing self-validation in genuine and helpful ways

Chapter **14**

Ten Tips for a Skillful Life

n this book, you have learned and, more importantly, practiced, many skills. However, practicing things once or twice does not make you skillful. For example, sitting at a keyboard once does not make you a piano player, or going to a French language class once does not make you a French speaker. When it comes to a life worth living, your desires and intentions will only get you so far. You need to continue to practice the skills you have learned on a regular basis to ensure that all aspects of your life have balance, and these aspects include your mental health, relationships, career, and so on. This chapter discusses ten practical tips for building on all you have learned in this book.

Periodically Review Your Short- and Long-Term Goals

Reviewing your goals regularly is crucial for staying on track, maintaining motivation, and making adjustments as needed. Use Worksheet 14-1 to review your goals.

Worksheet 14-1 My Goals

Identify your goals, both short- and long-term. Before you can review how you are doing, it is obviously important to know what your goals are. Write down your short-term goals and a few of your long-term goals.

_____

_____

_____

_____

_____

_____

Goals drive commitment. Keep your goals in mind and close to your heart.

Review the progress you have made toward attaining your goals. There will be times when life and its challenges make it more difficult to stay on the path toward attaining your goals, and at times, it will be easier. The key is not to give up when times are hard and to be kind to yourself when you fall short. If you have succeeded, celebrate your achievement! If you have a network of support, you can ask them for help or troubleshoot what went wrong. Review your goals and write down the progress you have made toward attaining them.

_____

_____

_____

_____

Write down any difficulties that have slowed your progress.

_____

_____

_____

_____

_____

Write down some possible solutions to your obstacles or the names of people who could help.

_____

_____

Make sure that your goals continue to align with your values. Write down your goals and your values and identify how they align. For instance, "My goal is to become a nurse," and "My values include helping people."

_____

_____

_____

Assess what's working: When we struggle, we tend to think about all the things that are not working. However, in many situations, there are many things that are working. Your life may have some failures but you also have many successes. What are the things that are working in your life? Write down some of the ways in which you are not struggling and the things that you are doing that are effective.

_____

_____

_____

_____

(continued)

Worksheet 14-1 *(continued)*

Make adjustments as needed. Be open to adjusting your goals based on new information, changing circumstances, or shifts in priorities. For instance, you may be wanting to complete a college degree but you have a baby on the way. What are some options? Could you study part-time? Can you take a deferral? Have your life circumstances changed, and if so how? It is also possible that your goal is now no longer relevant or achievable. Are there ways that you can modify or replace your goal with one that is more relevant to your new situation?

_____

_____

_____

_____

Never Stop Learning

In Chapter 7, on emotion regulation, you read about the ABC PLEASE skill, where the B is building mastery. You can go beyond building mastery and continuing to challenge and educate your mind and keep learning. Consider these tips:

>> **Take a class.** Many communities have continuing education or personal enrichment courses. Go online and type "continuing education," "personal enrichment," or "adult education" into a search tool, and you'll find many courses. Ask yourself what you would like to learn. Maybe you can find an interesting course over a long weekend or one that has weekly classes.

>> **Join a club.** Maybe you've wanted to learn how to ballroom dance, become better at yoga, or learn how to knit. Perhaps there is a book club hosted by your local book club. Name some things you'd like to learn or do with a group.

Practice Wholistic Health

Wholistic health includes healthy exercise, eating, and sleep. Almost every article, podcast, and TV show on living a healthy life includes recommendations on balanced eating, sleep, and exercise. We recognize that it is easier said than done. Here are some tips to sticking to your commitments and building the blocks of wholistic health.

Regular exercise

Exercise ideas:

>> **Open your calendar for the next three months.** If that feels like too much, do it for the next month. Ideally, you would exercise four or five times per week for 30 minutes. If you haven't exercised in a while, any regular exercise is better than none. If you can find time to exercise before or after work, that's great. If you can only workout on weekends, do it. Record the days when you have at least 30 minutes to work out, and note the time of day reserved for working out.

>> **Consider the type of exercise.** There are so many types of exercises, and there is always something you can do. Of course, the more you enjoy an exercise, the more you are likely to do it. There are low-impact exercises like walking and swimming, high-intensity exercises like cross training, exercises that you can do if you are injured, such as static exercises using the non-affected muscles, group exercises like yoga and Pilates, and so on. Pick one that you can commit to. Later, if you want to join a gym, you can, but for now, the goal is simply to move.

>> **Find a workout partner.** Even if you start, it can be difficult to persist. One way to persist is to be accountable to an exercise partner. Most people have someone in their life who is willing to exercise with them. Write down people you can reach out to, and see if they will join you in exercise and hold you accountable to your commitment.

TIP

>> **Eskew excuses.** Finally, don't let excuses become your mortal enemy. When it feels hard to stick to your commitment, it can be easy to say things like: "I'll do it tomorrow," "I'm too tired," "The new season of my favorite show is ready to binge," and so on. Write down the excuses you are most likely to use and commit to yourself or your exercise buddy to avoid excuses. Record the excuses that are most likely to show up.

Balanced diet

Consider these balanced eating ideas:

>> **Record your current diet.** Balanced eating is not about deprivation or any of the many named diets. It is about ensuring that your body gets the right amount of calories, minerals, vitamins, healthy fats, and proteins. The first thing to do is to write down your daily food intake.

Do I eat the same thing every day: Y/N

My protein source is: _____

My fruits and vegetables are: _____

My indulgence foods are: _____

>> **Clean out your pantry.** If your diet is not balanced, and your fridge or pantry is full of high calorie, low nutrition foods, it is time to do a deep cleanse of your fridge and pantry. Anything that is high in added sugar, trans fats, high-fructose corn syrup, or ingredients you can't pronounce are likely better in the trash than in your body. Take an inventory of these foods and throw them out. If it feels too drastic, first go healthy food shopping, and then

replace the less healthy food with your purchases. If you want to keep some of your indulgent food, keep a small amount. Record the list of food you are throwing out and then write down the list of the replacement items.

>> **Be mindful of your eating.** As highlighted throughout the book, mindfulness is the core skill of DBT. It is important for you to track how you feel and experience life after every intervention. No skill or recommendation is an instant and enduring solution. This is no less true with balanced eating.

Write down how you feel after the food changes that you make. You can track this daily or weekly.

Good sleeping habits

This section discusses ideas for developing better sleeping habits.

Start by recording your current sleep behavior. For many people who have a difficult time sleeping, a sleeping pill should often be the last resort. You can make many other changes to your sleep behavior that can dramatically improve your amount and quality of sleep. The first step is to make a map of your sleep behavior. Answer the following questions and reflect on whether your pattern of sleep is regular (even if it's poor) or irregular:

>> I drink caffeinated beverages before going to sleep: Y/N

>> I get in bed at (time): _____

>> I fall asleep immediately: Y/N

>> I use phone/tablet/TV screens when I am in bed before I fall asleep: Y/N

>> My room is dark at night: Y/N

>> The temperature in my room is on the cooler side: Y/N

>> I wake up frequently during the night: Y/N

>> I have frequent nightmares: Y/N

>> I wake up early in the morning, before I want to: Y/N

>> I can sleep all day: Y/N

>> I take frequent naps: Y/N

>> I feel rested after I sleep: Y/N

Write down the impact of your sleep quality. How do you feel after a good night's sleep versus after a poor night's sleep? Does this affect your mood? Your eating habits? Your productivity? Your relationships with others?

Make changes. Now that you have a better map of your sleep habits, try to change the ones that are clearly contributing to poor sleep, such as stimulant medication at night or caffeinated drinks before bedtime. Now commit to keep a consistent sleep routine.

>> I commit to be in bed by: _____ and wake up by _____.

Stick to a routine. Go to bed at the same time every night. If you choose to deviate from the plan, such as during a night out with friends, make sure that the pros outweigh the cons.

TIP

Ensure the temperature is conducive to sleeping. Research shows that the ideal room temperature for sleep is between 60 and 67° F. Above 67 and sleep quality deteriorates. If it's a cool evening out, considering leaving your window open. Considering using a fan or any air-conditioner or sleeping under fewer blankets.

Sleep in a dark room. If you have excess light in your room coming from electronic devices, remove these. If you have a playlist on your phone that helps you sleep, have the playlist on a timer and make sure it's truly soothing. After you have set your morning alarm, make sure that the phone is on airplane mode and away from your bed. Resist the temptation to pick it up and start scrolling your news or social media feeds.

Avoid going to bed on a full stomach. It may not be completely obvious, but large meals and alcohol can affect the quality of sleep. Even if you sleep enough hours, you might not get into a state of deep sleep. If dinner is your main meal of the day, make sure to have it on the earlier side of the evening and not right before climbing into bed.

Limit Drugs and Alcohol

This workbook is not focused on substance use, but you cannot have a skillful life if substances are impacting your psychological and physical health. This is not about stopping drug and alcohol use altogether. The task here is to consider the impact that drugs and alcohol are having in your life.

>> What impact are drugs and alcohol having in your life? Write down the impact on your psychological, physical, occupational, academic, and relational life.

>> What is keeping your drug and alcohol use going? What is reinforcing the behavior? Are you using the substances to connect with others? To change how you feel? Because you like them?

>> What is the routine of your substance use? When do use your drugs or alcohol? How many days a week? Who do you use with?

>> Now that you have answered all these questions, and you see the impact on your life, consider the specific changes you can make to modify and ideally reduce your use.

Limit News and Social Media

Have you ever had food poisoning or stomach issues because of something you ate? Do you feel better after certain foods and worse after others? What you ingest matters. Think about social media and your newsfeed the same way. They are food sources for your brain. Pay attention to how they impact you. You may notice that some social media and newsfeeds make you sick with depression, anxiety, and despair. Others make you happy. If you notice that you feel worse after ingesting today's news and social media, consider these tips for modifying your use consistent with a value-driven and skillful life:

- » **Set clear boundaries.** If you are spending endless hours on social medial or your news-feed, and this is making you more depressed or anxious, it may be a matter of the dose or quantity that your brain is consuming. Commit to a designated amount of time per day and a time of day when you allow yourself to use social media. In particular, if you feel worse at night, commit to not use it then. Use a timer to indicate when the time is up.

- » **Remove temptation.** If there are certain social media apps that make you feel particularly bad, delete them from your phone or move them to a separate folder, where they are less accessible. If this step is too steep, turn off notifications for those particular apps. Review the apps on your phone and divide them into ones that bring you joy, ones that are neutral, and ones that make you feel worse about yourself. Can you delete them right now? You are on your way to become a DBT superstar if you can do it right now.

- » **Replace social media time with other activities.** Go back to Chapter 7, the emotion regulation skills, and review your ABC PLEASE skills. Focus on the accumulating positives and building mastery skills. Use these skills as ways to fill the time you would normally spend on social media. For instance, you could be reading, cooking, gardening, exercising, playing music, learning a new language, meditating, and many other things.

- » **Use technology tools and apps.** It may seem odd to use technology tools to reduce your technology use, but features like the Do Not Disturb mode on your phone can help minimize distractions. These are particularly helpful when you are sleeping, eating, working, or out with friends,.

- » **Create physical barriers.** Designate certain areas of your home as social media-free zones, where you don't use your device. Research shows that being on social media or being distracted while driving increases your risk of an accident, even more than being on substances. Commit to not checking your phone while driving. Put your cell phone in the back seat of the car until you get home, or if you have to have it on you, commit to pulling over before checking your notifications. If you are a parent, you are also modeling healthier behavior for your kids.

- » **Reflect on your goals.** It's important to remind yourself about *why* you want to reduce your social media usage. Is it to improve focus? Improve your mental health or your relationships? Be more productive? Keep your goals in mind. One activity that can help is to buy a journal and track your progress.

Be Accountable to Others

Holding yourself accountable to others is another way of establishing and maintaining a skillful life, because it helps to create a sense of trust and reliability. When people know they can count on you, they'll be more inclined to want to help you when you are struggling. Here are some ideas:

>> **Share your goals with the supportive people in your life.** Communicate your specific goals and plans to friends, family, a mentor, or your therapist. Ideally include timelines and actions steps. This has two main benefits — when others are aware of what you're working toward, they can offer you support and encouragement. It can be an adaptive use of the emotion of guilt, knowing how you will feel if you let others down. Write down the names of the people who you can ask to hold you accountable.

>> **Set up regular progress reviews.** It might help to reach out to the people you have just identified, the ones who will hold you accountable, and schedule check-ins to discuss your progress. This will be a more helpful recommendation for longer-term plans, but you can certainly use check-ins for shorter-term goals, such gym membership, signing up for classes, speaking to a person you have been avoiding, and so on.

>> **Join a graduate support group.** Some people, after they have completed DBT treatment, find that having a community of others who have gone through DBT is a supportive experience. Some DBT practices offer advanced or graduate DBT groups. There is nothing stopping you from forming your own group with some of your co-graduates.

>> **Implement your own set of rewards and consequences.** Many people who come to DBT tend to self-invalidate by thinking they "should" be able to do certain things, given that most people they know can do those things. Or, they feel that they don't deserve to be rewarded. This type of thinking is not compassionate.

TIP

Do nice things for yourself when you have attained something you were aiming for — something that has been difficult for you. The rewards need not be big. Treat yourself to a bubble bath, a nice meal out, or some leisure time. Similarly, you can set up consequences for not completing something you had committed to. However, this should *not* be a punishment, but something that will keep you on track. For instance, if you have a project or term paper due, and you had considered going out with friends, maybe you decide you can't go out with them until your project is complete. Write down some ways in which you can reward yourself for completing your short-term goals. Also, write down meaningful and non-punitive consequences for not completing your commitments. Make sure these consequences are aligned with your values and ones that can help you stay on track.

Accumulate Positives

Accumulating positives is a skill from the emotion regulation skillset and targets the elements that make you vulnerable to painful emotions. Adding and accumulating positives in your life is a great way to create a wall between you and the suffering caused by emotional overload.

>> **Commit to doing one pleasant thing every day.** Positive events are the ones you find pleasurable or bring you joy. Your task is to do these without feeling guilty that you are indulging yourself. You are indulging yourself and yet, in all likelihood, you have suffered a lot, so you deserve some good things in your life. Create a list of things that bring you joy (even in small measures!) and commit to practice at least one each day. Try to add as many to the list as you can. Examples might include taking a nap, eating your favorite snack, getting a massage, taking a bubble bath, buying an item that you've wanted, and so on.

» **While accumulating positives, try to do so mindfully.** You might think that there is nothing positive in your life. Your task is to enjoy your enjoyable moments when you are experiencing them and highlight the difference between pleasant moments and painful ones.

» **Be unmindful of worrying.** In this context, we are prescribing mindLESSness! Don't pollute your positive experiences with worrying or thinking about when the positive experiences will end.

» **Reflect on your day and consider some of the good things that happened.** If you are someone who likes to journal, you can also write down any positive events or interactions that you experienced.

» **Don't avoid.** One of the ways of delaying the impact of the positives in your life is to procrastinate from doing the things that need to get done. Sometimes, the things that need to get done aren't ones that bring you joy. For instance, if you have to address trauma in therapy, you know that this will likely be painful, and yet by avoiding doing the work that needs to get done, it will always be at the back of your mind and will impact your experience of joyful moments.

Build Mastery

Building mastery, which is under the emotion regulation skill of DBT, is core to creating a skillful life, because it entails connecting or reconnecting with our drive to feel competent, and in so doing, create a sense of accomplishment and possibly even pride. See Worksheet 14-2.

Worksheet 14-2   Building Mastery

The first step is to decide what you want to build mastery in. If you are not musically inclined or have no ear for it, learning to play the violin is probably not a great choice. On the other hand, if you always wanted to learn to paint, speak a new language, or play a new sport, these are activities that you might build mastery on. Write down something that you have always wanted to do, but never had the time or opportunity to do.

_____

_____

_____

_____

Next, consider whether you have the time, finances, and expert resources to learn the thing that you want to learn. For instance, if you want to learn tennis, are there tennis courts nearby? If you want to learn to play chess, is there a chess teacher in your neighborhood? If you want to learn to cook, do you have the financial resources to pay for the classes and all the ingredients you will need to buy? Also, remember that many classes can be taken online, although some are better done in-person.

>> Is the thing that I want to build mastery in available to me in terms of geographical proximity and expertise? Y/N

>> Can I take the course online or using an app?

>> If I am going to have to pay for it, is it expensive? Can I afford to pay the teacher and pay for the raw ingredients, tools, or materials that I may have to buy? Y/N

>> If I have the time, the place, the teacher, and the resources to take on the challenge of building mastery, when can I start? Go online and find out if you have to sign up for classes or if you can follow the instructions of an online course.

>> What is my cope ahead plan if I start to lose interest or am finding things too difficult? Write down your cope ahead plan.

_____

_____

_____

_____

_____

Use the Coping Ahead Skill

Coping ahead is the skill of making a plan for when things don't go as you thought they would. By the time you have reached this section of the book and if you have been in DBT therapy, you'll be very familiar with the cope ahead skill. This section is less about coping ahead in crisis situations and more about the practice of coping ahead with everyday challenges. Try these steps:

1. **Write down the thing that you are worried about.** Think about the thing that might causes stress if it does happen or that causes you distress if it does not happen. For instance, "I am worried that I will fail a test," "I am worried that I won't get the job I applied for," "I am worried that I will be picked to give a presentation."

2. **Write down your concerns should your fear come to pass.** Be clear about the worst thing that could happen. Write down the feelings you anticipate will show up.

3. **Write down what you are going to do if the worst happens**. Make sure you're specific about your plans to cope with this scenario.

4. **Rehearse the worst-case scenario over and over in your head.** Ideally, the rehearsal practice should also induce the emotions associated with the situation. The goal is to fully imagine the situation, including the emotions you will feel should it happen. Now, go back to the plan in Step 3 and rehearse it until you have the plan set in your mind.

Practice Flexibility

Psychological flexibility is when you are able to stay fully present even when you are struggling with negative thoughts and emotions *and* choose behaviors that are driven by your values rather your moods. Psychological flexibility is powerfully associated with quality of life and mental well-being. Try these steps:

1. **The first step to attaining psychological flexibility is being willing to feel difficult emotions.** Many people who are in DBT treatment know what painful emotions are and often want to avoid them. Avoidance of suffering leads to more suffering.

2. **Next, you have to practice learning how to step back from your thoughts.** This means distancing the content of your thoughts from believing that they are true. Write down the content of the thoughts you have and then write down whether you believe them to be true, independent of any data. For instance, "I have the thought that no one loves me," and "I believe this to be true."

3. **Next, focus on the present moment.** Focus on what is. Write down the thoughts that you have that are present moment thoughts. Write down thoughts that plague you about the past, and then write down the worries that you have about the future.

4. **Connect rather than comparing.** We all want to belong, and our task is to connect with the people we love. However, when we feel threatened, we tend to focus on all the things that we don't have and are envious of all the things that others have. Rather than focusing on connecting, we slip into comparisons.

   Write down all the ways that you compare your situation to others and, in particular, the comparisons that leave you feeling worse about yourself. Next, write down the people who you feel you have lost connection with and write down the reasons that have interfered with strengthening those connections.

Chapter **15**

Ten Ways to Overcome Obstacles

O bstacles are part of life. They show up both in and out of therapy. One of the challenging things about when you hit an obstacle is that you can experience strong emotions. Those strong emotions can stop you in your tracks and, at worst, lead to you abandoning your goals.

The good news is that you can learn to anticipate and plan for obstacles as well as navigate them in the moment. In this book, you have learned many DBT skills that help you tackle the obstacles in your way and the emotions that accompany them.

Anticipate Obstacles When You Can

Anticipating obstacles helps you be less emotionally vulnerable. Use your cope ahead skill from the ABC PLEASE skill (see Chapter 7) to cope ahead for obstacles when you can. Anticipating things that can get in your way and making a plan for them will help you move forward with more confidence. Remember, when you anticipate obstacles, you are considering that things might not going as planned and the emotions that may that. This will give you the opportunity to think about how you can manage both the obstacle and the feelings that may arise, as well as think about the next steps.

Validate the Emotions that Show Up

Validating your emotions helps you understand your experience and grab control of your emotions. Obstacles can lead to dysregulation and interfere with your ability to accurately assess the situation, as well as think about how you can effectively navigate it. You need to be regulated before you can be reflective or problem solve, and self-validation helps you get your thinking back online and make a wise decision about what to do next.

Remember to Breathe

Remember to breathe! Some people who are emotionally sensitive have been told to take a deep breath in ways that feel invalidating. If that has happened to you, we are hoping to change your relationship with your breath. You breathe all the time, and mostly you do this automatically and mindlessly. One of your most powerful tools to help you regulate your emotions is your breath. Just three mindful breaths can help slow down your thoughts and calm your physiology. If it is helpful to practice a specific way to breathe, you can use the paced breathing from your TIPP skill (see Chapter 9) to ensure that your out breath is longer than your in breath. Try inhaling for a count of six and exhaling for a count of eight.

Keep Your Goal in Mind

Keeping your ultimate goal in mind, even when you hit an obstacle, can be a great motivator. It is easy to experience disappointment, fear, anger, and other emotions when you run into an obstacle and then forget your goal or suddenly feel like it is no longer important.

REMEMBER

Emotionally sensitive people can struggle with mood-dependent behaviors (see Chapter 12) and lose sight of their goals in the face of strong emotions. Use strategies to remember what you are hoping for as you approach situations. Sticking to your goals and persevering will give you a sense of mastery and confidence that will serve you well from that time onward.

Practice Effectiveness

Practicing your mindfulness effectiveness skill is stepping back and doing what the situation calls for (see Chapter 6). It is remembering your goals while also taking into account what is going on around you. Being effective is always helpful when you come upon an obstacle. Remember your goal and also step back and assess what is happening in front of you right now. By being effective, you can see what needs to happen next, and then pivot if you need to while staying on track with the goal you have in mind.

Understand the Problem

All too often, we try to solve problems before we understand the exact nature of the problem. When you encounter an obstacle, slow down and try to understand what happened. Start by assessing the problem. Think about what happened. Next, define the obstacle or problem. Once you have defined it, consider what caused the problem. Stay open minded and stick to the facts. It is important to avoid making assumptions. Once you understand the obstacle or problem, make an action plan. Now that you have a plan, move ahead with it, which will help you get back on track.

Engage in Problem Solving

DBT teaches five ways to address a problem. To navigate the problem that may be getting in your way, you can use any of these problem-solving strategies. The acronym to help you remember these five problem-solving strategies is SCREW:

- **Solve the problem:** The best way to address a problem is to solve it. If you can solve the problem, then you should; however, it is not always easy or even possible to solve the problem at all or in the timeframe you would like. For this reason, there are four other options.

- **Change the relationship:** When you can't solve the problem, find a way to change your relationship to the problem, which can change how you feel about it. Try to find a silver lining or, as Dr Linehan says, make lemonade out of lemons.

- **Radically accept:** Sometimes, you may have to choose to radically accept and tolerate the problem as it is. Let go of judgement, accept it, and see how you can work with it exactly as it is.

- **Entertain misery:** You can always stay miserable. Staying miserable for a short time can be validating; however, be mindful of not getting stuck in misery, which leads to suffering.

- **Worsen the problem:** Although it is not ideal, you can always make the problem worse. The goal here is to be mindful when you are heading in this direction, so you can catch yourself and engage in a more effective type of problem solving.

It is helpful to remember that when you encounter an obstacle that feels like a problem you cannot solve, there are other ways you can address it.

Ask for Help If You Need It

Asking for help is a skill that we all need; however, it is easier for some people than for others. When you hit an obstacle, asking for help can sometimes be the key to getting unstuck. Other people can provide validation and ideas that you can't always see in the moment.

Be effective when you ask for help. Make sure that you are clear about what you are asking. Remember to ask for what you need so that the other person can be most helpful. Let the other person know when you want the help and make sure what you are asking for is realistic and doable.

If you have difficulty asking for help, it is an incredible skill to practice. Remember that asking for help can build connections and help you learn new ways to approach a problem. There is also wonderful data that helping another person promotes feelings of happiness, increased self-esteem, and even changes in psychology like lower blood pressure. If you struggle with asking for help, make this practice a habit. The more you practice asking for help, the easier it will become.

Pivot If You Need To

Sometimes, you need to change your plan. In these cases, the most effective approach to an obstacle may be to practice radical acceptance (see Chapter 9) and be open to pivoting and changing your plan. Changing course can be challenging, as you must take a deep breath and let go of any attachment you have to your plan. When you pivot, make sure you validate the feelings that arise. You will likely have to give up something you were hoping for, like a specific outcome or a timeframe.

Use Encouragement to Stay in the Process

Effective self-encouragement can help you maintain motivation and perseverance when things get difficult. Many people who come to DBT have difficulty with encouragement because they struggle with self-loathing or self-hatred. Using effective encouragement can help you achieve goals as well as navigate big challenges like obstacles.

Developing ways to encourage yourself can take time. Think about how you would encourage yourself to keep going in a difficult situation, such as running a marathon on a hot day. What could you say to yourself? These statements do not have to be elaborate, they just have to be meaningful to you. Consider simple statements like: "I've got this," "I can do hard things," "Do the next thing," or "I have the skills, strength, or ability to do this." Or, as Dory says, "Just keep swimming!"

IN THIS CHAPTER

» Considering the value of
   self-validation

» Recognizing when you are not
   validating your feelings

» Taking the steps to self-validate

Chapter **16**

Ten Ways to Self-Validate

In the first few chapters, you learned how being emotionally sensitive combined with chronic invalidation can lead to significant problems in regulation of mood, relationships, thoughts, and behaviors. When people have been invalidated by their environment, they often continue invalidating themselves as a response to their own emotions, which can be just as painful and unhelpful. Of course, it is comforting to get validation from others, but you can't always count on it. The most powerful form of validation is self-validation.

REMEMBER

Any time you find yourself saying things like: "I shouldn't feel this way," "I should just get over it," "I am overreacting," or "I should have known what to do," you are likely self-invalidating.

The Benefits of Self-Validation

Once you develop self-validation as a skill, you will see its power and recognize that it is enduring and not dependent on other people. Self-validation is the recognition and acceptance that your internal and private experiences — whether emotions, thoughts, or behaviors — are valid. Your ability to validate your own experience is an important step in establishing and strengthening your self-worth, your abilities, and your successes. It also helps you soothe and regulate painful emotions. It's hard to validate yourself initially, and it is understandable to want others to validate and recognize you. However, when you can do this on your own, you will notice a greater sense of freedom and self-worth.

Remember, self-validation:

>> **Boosts your self-esteem and your confidence:** You are acknowledging your self-worth and your potential and strengthening your self-esteem as a consequence, and once you are practiced, your confidence in your abilities will bloom and grow.

>> **Promotes emotional resilience and wellbeing:** Having to rely on others to tell you how to feel and how to act on those feelings makes you very dependent on them. Of course, it's wonderful to have a supportive group of people on your side, but they might not always be around. Self-validation helps you build emotional resilience by teaching you how to cope and rely on your own judgment when times are difficult. When you acknowledge and accept your feelings as valid, you feel better. You are also able to express your feelings effectively, and you won't need to resort to excessive displays of emotions or suppressing, denying, or avoiding them.

>> **Helps regulate your emotions:** Validating your emotions helps you stay with the primary emotion (which are fleeting), rather than potentially escalating the suffering with secondary emotions, as noted in Chapter 7.

Ten Steps to Validation

Here are the ten steps necessary to self-validate.

1. **Be willing to practice self-validation.** Willingness is the readiness and agreement to practice self-validation. It is the willingness to say that what you are feeling is valid. You believe that it makes sense that — given your genetics, temperament, biology, and environmental experiences — you would feel the way you do and behave the way you do.

   Rather than judging your emotional responses, are you willing to practice self-validation and throw yourself wholeheartedly into doing so?

   _____

2. **Acknowledge that the feeling or behavior is there.** Once you have agreed to practicing self-validation, you next have to acknowledge your feelings, thoughts, and behaviors. Rejecting these is falling back into self-invalidation. Acknowledgement includes the act of putting a name to the emotion, thought, or behavior, such as: "I am feeling sad," "I think people don't like me," or "I yelled at my co-worker." Acknowledgement includes the act of labeling.

   Think about a situation that has triggered a strong emotional and behavioral response. Can you acknowledge what happened? Describe the situation.

   _____

   _____

_____

_____

3. **Accept your feelings and thoughts.** Once you acknowledge the feelings, you have to accept them. It is important not to equate accepting feelings with liking feelings. If you have a severe toothache, accepting that it is there does not mean that you have to like it. But if you keep taking pain killers and refusing to accept the pain, the problem will become much worse. The same thing happens with emotions.

   Think about the situation in Step 2. You have acknowledged that your emotions and thoughts were present. Can you accept them? Write down what you are accepting and make a distinction between accepting and liking your emotion or response.

   _____

   _____

   _____

   _____

4. **Allow the feelings to be there without avoiding them or trying to escape from them.** Almost no one likes feeling painful emotions, and it is understandable that you would want to get as far away from them as you can. Avoiding or trying to escape them actually ends up doing the opposite of what you want, which is to be able to self-validate and manage the feelings.

   Allow the feelings to be there. This is a key practice and is consistent with learning and behavioral theory. When a child learns to swim, they are often initially afraid of the water and cling to the side of the pool or stay close to their parent or teacher. Over time, they realize that the water is not as terrifying as they imagined it to be. The same is true of emotions. The more you experience them and allow them to "be" without trying to fight or modify them, the more you can observe them as phenomena that rise and fall and the more dominion you will have over them.

   Allowing the feelings includes the following types of statements:

   - This is the way I feel right now.

   - It is not wrong that I am having this emotion right now.

   - Allowing myself to feel this way doesn't mean that I have to behave in any specific way.

   - Nothing stays the same, and this emotion will pass, but for now this emotion is here.

   - This emotion is uncomfortable, and I don't like it, but the emotion itself can't hurt me.

Recall a situation that caused you some strong emotion and, in particular, an emotion you tried hard to avoid. Allow for the feeling to arise and to simply be there. Write down what happens to the feeling as you experience it, then write down statements that recognize that the feeling is present and that it will pass.

_____

_____

_____

_____

_____

_____

5. **Understand your experience, given your past.** You have accepted that you are having the feelings or emotions that you are having. But where did they come from? Feelings and emotions make sense given your emotional sensitivity and things that happened in your past. For example, say that you have been bitten by a dog more than once in your life. You are walking around with your friend who says, "Look at that cute puppy!" Fear shows up inside of you. If you remember dialectics, it makes sense that your friend is not afraid of puppy dogs, AND (the dialectical AND) it also makes sense that you are afraid of puppies. So, your experience of fear is understandable, given your past.

Think about an emotion that tends to show up frequently and then reflect on the events that happened in the past that elicited similar emotional responses.

_____

_____

_____

_____

6. **Understand your experience, given your present.** Many times, the reason you are feeling a strong emotion is less about what happened in the past and more about what is happening in the present moment. For example, let's say that you have a dear colleague at work or classmate at school. You two are very close, and that colleague or classmate is not particularly close to anyone else. They announce that they are being transferred to a new job or moving to a new school, and you feel devastated. No one else is upset at all. This is where you need to self-validate given your present circumstances. The person that you have grown close to is leaving. Given your relationship, it makes perfect sense that you would feel sad, and that no one else would.

Think about persistent thoughts and intense emotions that you are presently experiencing, given an event that is going on right now in your life. Write down the thoughts and emotions and reflect on how they make sense. Remember not to judge the thoughts or emotions, nor tell yourself that you should not be feeling the way you are feeling.

_____

_____

_____

_____

_____

7. **Troubleshoot your self-validation.** For many people who are just beginning the process of practicing self-validation, just like any new skill, it can feel as if it is simply too difficult. Just like any other difficulties and lack of skill that you might have, the difficulty of practicing self-validation is precisely why this skill is so important. At first, as you head down the path of self-validation, your mind and emotions will turn to all the painful emotions and negative ways of thinking that tell you that you can't do it. It will be difficult when you try to switch "I can't do this" to "I know that this is a new skill for me, and that it will be difficult at first, but I need to persist." By being patient with yourself, you are practicing a form of compassionate, self-validation, and then as with all skills, it will become easier the more you practice it.

Think about what gets in the way of self-validation. Are you not practicing it regularly enough for it to be a habit? Do you feel that you are lying to yourself? Do you feel that you can't do it? All of these are typical problems in overcoming self-validation.

What are the thoughts or emotions that get in the way of your self-validation, and what can you do to remind yourself to practice? Again, it is very important that you not judge your thoughts or emotions, or you tell yourself that you should not be feeling the way you are feeling.

_____

_____

_____

_____

_____

8. **Realize that it makes sense to self-invalidate.** Almost everyone who self-invalidates learned to do so when they were young. You may have been told to not get upset, that you are making a big deal over nothing, that you should stop complaining, or that you have it better than others. Your initial reactions are not choices. You don't wake up in the morning and decide that you are going to make your life or someone else's life miserable. Simply being told that you are overreacting is hurtful, when you don't know how to react.

   Imagine that you had a severe case of poison ivy. People would never tell you that you are making a big deal over nothing, you should just get over it, or that others have it better than you do. Clearly, a poison ivy rash is visible to others, but your private experiences are not.

   However, YOU are the one who knows how you feel. If you realize that your automatic response is to self-invalidate, all you are doing is repeating the hurtful commentary of your past, and this makes sense, especially if it was all you heard. Self-invalidation is not the healthiest way to deal with how you feel.

   Take a reaction that you commonly have and one that you tend to respond to with self-invalidation. Write down how it makes sense that you self-invalidate. Write that statement down three times, and then highlight how your self-invalidation statements have become automatic.

   _____

   _____

   _____

   _____

9. **The truth is NOT self-invalidation, so do not validate what is not true.** If something is a fact, it is simply a fact, whether you like it or not. Reality does not change itself to your liking. Let's say that you are not good at tennis. Saying "I am bad at tennis" is a

fact and is not self-invalidating. You might want to modify the statement to, "I have no talent in tennis," rather than saying you are bad at it.

Now, say that you are talented at writing. You are in college or at work and have to write up a report. You typically produce outstanding work, but this report is not your best. Making statements like, "I am stupid," "I am a terrible writer," or "I should quit and find something else to do," ARE self-invalidating statements because you are filtering your entire experience, one with great results, through the lens of one less-than-stellar result. Saying "I am stupid" is self-invalidating, but saying "I am not good at tennis" is not. Nor would you say, "I am great at tennis," as this would be validating something that is not true and therefore, not valid.

Say you do poorly on a test and say, "I did poorly on that test, and so I am stupid." It is valid that you did poorly on the test, you have the result to prove it. It is not valid to say that you are stupid, and you could certainly assess what the conditions were that caused you to do poorly on the test.

Or say that your partner tells you that you are texting them too many times while they are at work, and they are finding it disruptive to their workflow. Saying, "My partner is finding it disruptive that I text so much, they find me annoying, and want to break up with me," has a valid statement — that you are texting too often while they are at work — and an invalid statement — that they find it annoying and want to break up with you. If your partner said that you were annoying them, it would be valid to say that they find the behavior annoying, but without them saying so, concluding that you are annoying is simply your interpretation.

Write down a statement that reflects your self-invalidation. Is there any truth to the statement? You want to discern the elements that are self-invalidating and those that are not. Write down the invalid elements and the valid ones. Remember that valid statements are fact-based, with evidence, and not simply valid because you think they are true.

_____

_____

_____

_____

10. **Consider your future-self.** Your future needs you, and your past does not. If you continue to self-invalidate now, your future-self will do this as well. Practicing self-validation now will allow your future-self to be far better at self-validation.

Think about a future you a few years from now, looking back at you today. You are either disappointed that you continued to self-invalidate or are proud for changing the narrative of self-invalidation. You can describe the aspiring future-self, or if you are an artist, you can draw future-you talking to present-you.

_____

_____

_____

Index

A

ABC PLEASE skill
  ABC portion, 140–141
  overview, 140
  PLEASE portion, 140–142
  worksheets, 143–145
abilities of future self, 279
acceptance
  ACCEPTS skill, 181–182
  change and, 16–19
  practices to help with, 197
  radical, practicing, 193–196
  turning the mind, 196
  willingness and willfulness, 197–199
Accepting Admirable Qualities worksheet, 278
ACCEPTS skill, 181–182
accountability, 292–293
accumulating positives, 293–294
active passivity, 222–223, 228–230
activities, 181
adolescents, typical versus problematic behaviors in, 215–217
alcohol abuse
  behavioral dysregulation, 31–32
  commitment to change, 59–60
  crisis kit, 199–200
  limiting, 291
  PLEASE skills, 142
  risky behaviors, 271–273
  sources of suffering, 45
all-or-nothing thinking, 88–89, 118
AND
  depolarizing experiences using, 18
  generating dialectical thinking using, 205–206
anger, 136, 139, 175–176
Answers worksheet, 177
anticipating obstacles, 297
apparent competence, 222–223, 230–232
asking for help, 299–300
Assessing Typical Adolescent Behaviors worksheet, 216–217

assumptions, 19–20
attachment, letting go of, 76–81
autonomy, forcing, 210–212

B

balanced eating, 142, 289–290
barriers
  to DBT therapy, 63–64
  due mental health conditions, 62
  to effectiveness in relationships, 62
  to emotion regulation, 63
  to mindfulness, 62, 131–132
  overcoming, 64–67
  overview, 61–63
  to radical acceptance, 194
behavior substitution, 32
behavioral dysregulation, 10, 13, 31–33, 40
behaviorism, 21, 98
behaviors. *See also* mood-dependent behaviors
  being behaviorally specific, 49–52
  extinction and, 99–102
  functions of, 96–97
  opposite actions, 100
  overview, 95
  principles of, 95–96
  punishments, effective and ineffective, 105–106
  reinforcers, 98–102
  risky, 274–276
  self-reinforcement, 103–104
  shaping, 103–104
  typical versus problematic adolescent behaviors, 215–216
Being Behaviorally Specific worksheet, 51–52
biosocial theory, 21–22, 28
Borderline Personality Disorder (BPD), 8–10
both/and, embracing, 90
breathing, 70–71, 187, 298
Building Mastery worksheet, 294–295

C

calm strips, 186

capabilities, enhancing with therapy, 23–24

catastrophizing, 118

Causes of Suffering in My Life worksheet, 45–46

challenging emotions, identifying, 150

change

   acceptance coexisting with, 16–19

   consequences of not committing to, 59–60

   encouraging patient to, 24

choices for therapy, 67

Clarifying My Short- and Long-Term Goals worksheet, 58–59

coexisting opposites, coping with, 17

cognitive distortions, 87, 118–119

cognitive dysregulation, 10, 13, 36–37, 40

commitment

   barriers to, 61–64

   causes of suffering, 44–46

   consequences of not changing, 59–60

   freedom of choice, 67

   goals and, 55–59

   I Am Fully Committed To. . ., 61

   importance of patient's perspective, 44

   Making a Choice worksheet, 67

   My Barriers to DBT Therapy worksheet, 63–64

   Past Accomplishments worksheet, 66

comparison skill, 181

competencies, identifying, 230–232

Components of My Crisis Kit worksheet, 201–202

compromises versus dialectics, 204–205

conflict, managing with THINK skill, 175–176

Considering My True Nature worksheet, 263

contribution skill, 181

coping ahead skill, 295–297

Coping with Coexisting Opposites worksheet, 17

crises situations, identifying, 232–235

crisis kit, 201–202

curiosity, 288

current behaviors, identifying, 262

D

dangerous behaviors

   driving, 270

   sexual, 267–268

DBT (Dialectical Behavior Therapy)

   assumptions about, 19–20

   components of, 25–26

   effectiveness, 68

   encouraging patient's motivation to change, 24

   enhancing therapist's motivation to treat people, 25

   modes and functions, 23–25

   origins of, 8–10

   overview, 7

   principles and protocols, 21–23

   structuring environment for treatment, 25

DBT Skills for Reaching My Future Self worksheet, 281–282

DEAR MAN skill, 155–159

dependence, fostering, 210–212

Depolarizing Experiences Using AND worksheet, 18

dialectical dilemmas

   active passivity, dealing with, 228–230

   active passivity versus apparent competence, 222–223

   apparent competence, dealing with, 230–232

   emotional vulnerability, dealing with, 225–226

   emotional vulnerability versus self-invalidation, 222

   Gratitude for the People No Longer in My Life worksheet, 237

   How my Emotions Are Impacted by Sleep Quality worksheet, 226

   inhibited grieving, dealing with, 235–237

   Losses I Have Experienced worksheet, 236

   middle path

      fostering dependency and forcing autonomy, 209–210

      too loose and too strict, 212–213

      typical versus problematic adolescent behaviors, 215–218

      Walking the Middle Path worksheet, 218–219

   My Crises Situations worksheet, 232–235

   My Experience of the Dialectical Dilemmas worksheet, 224

   My Negative Self-Talk and Negative Self-Judgments worksheet, 227–228

   My Physical Reactions to Emotions worksheet, 225–226

   My True Competencies worksheet, 230–232

   overview, 221–222

   paradoxes, embracing, 238–241

   Replacing Judgments with Observable Facts worksheet, 228

self-invalidation, dealing with, 226–228

Task at Hand worksheet, 229

unrelenting crises, dealing with, 232–235

unrelenting crisis versus inhibited grieving, 223

Ways to Embrace My Paradoxes worksheet, 241

dialectics

  acceptance and change, 16–19

  compromises versus, 204–205

  Coping with Coexisting Opposites worksheet, 17

  defined, 90

  Depolarizing Experiences Using AND worksheet, 18

  dialectical synthesis, 17

  Dialectical Thinking worksheet, 15–16

  Embracing Both/And worksheet, 90

  general discussion, 14–16

  Goal/No Goal, 56

  overview, 221

  practicing dialectical thinking, 206–208

Did These Hypotheses Generate Any New Emotions? worksheet, 97

disagreement, validation of, 165–166

disgust, 138

disqualifying the positive, 118

distress tolerance

  acceptance and, 193–196

  ACCEPTS skill, 181–182

  Components of My Crisis Kit worksheet, 201–202

  crisis kit, 199–202

  Diving into Encouragement worksheet, 184

  IMPROVE the Moment worksheet, 185

  It's Time to Use TIPP worksheet, 188

  My Barriers to Radical Acceptance worksheet, 194

  My Wise Mind ACCEPTS worksheet, 182

  overview, 179–180

  Practicing My Pros and Cons worksheet, 192

  Practicing Radical Acceptance worksheet, 195–196

  Practicing the STOP Skill worksheet, 189–190

  pros and cons, using, 190–192

  self-soothing skills, using, 185–186

  Self-Soothing Skills worksheet, 186

  Signs of My Willfulness worksheet, 198–199

  STOP skill, 188–190

  TIPP skill, 187–188

  "turning the mind" skill, 196–197

  willingness and willfulness, understanding, 197–198

Diving into Encouragement worksheet, 184

Do I Have Problems Controlling My Behaviors? worksheet, 32

Do I Have Problems Dealing with My Emotions? worksheet, 30

Do I Have Problems in Close Relationships? worksheet, 34–35

Do I Have Problems in How I Think? worksheet, 37

Do I Struggle with Knowing Who I Am and My Sense of Self? worksheet, 39

driving behaviors, dangerous, 270

drug abuse

  limiting, 291

  PLEASE skills, 142

  risky behaviors, 271–273

  sources of suffering, 45

dysregulation

  behavioral, 10, 13, 31–33, 40

  cognitive, 10, 13, 36–37, 40

  cycle, 40

  Dysregulation worksheet, 10–13

  emotional, 9–10, 28–30, 40

  overview, 27

  sense-of-self, 10, 12, 38–40

Dysregulation worksheet, 10–13

E

eating

  balanced, 142, 289–290

  harmful behaviors, 269

effectiveness, practicing, 129–130, 298

Embracing Both/And worksheet, 90

emotion mind, 111–112

emotional dysregulation, 9–10, 28–30, 40

emotional reactivity, 9

emotional reasoning, 118

emotional vulnerabilities

  ABC PLEASE inventory of current, 143

  dealing with, 225–226

  versus self-invalidation, 222

emotions
  ABC PLEASE Inventory of Current Emotional Vulnerabilities worksheet, 143
  ABC PLEASE Skills Weekly Tracking Reflections worksheet, 145
  ACCEPTS skill, 181
  calming, 110
  changing with opposite action, 148–150
  Did These Hypotheses Generate Any New Emotions? worksheet, 97
  eliminating decision making driven by, 255–257
  emotion mind, 111–112
  Emotional Reactivity worksheet, 9
  function of, 134
  identifying, 134–139, 150
  justified, 139
  naming, 142
  negative mood states, 29
  PLEASE Skills Red Flags and Reflection worksheet, 145
  Practicing Opposite Action worksheet, 151–152
  primary, 135–138
  regulating
    ABC PLEASE skill, 140–145
    benefits, 133–134
    overview, 139–140
    SUN WAVE NO NOT skill, 146–148
  sadness, 136
  secondary, 138–139
  sleep quality, impact on, 226
  SUN WAVE NO NOT worksheet, 147–148
  understanding one's, 134–139
  unjustified, 139
  validating, 298
  Weekly ABC PLEASE Tracking Sheet worksheet, 144
  What I Learned from My Emotions worksheet, 135
encouragement skill, 183–184, 300
envy, 137
exercise, 142, 187, 289
extinction, 99–102

F

FAST skills, 169–173
fear, 137, 213–214
flexibility, psychological, 296
forcing autonomy, 210–212
former self, 262–263
fortune telling, 118

fostering dependence, 210–212
future self
  Accepting Admirable Qualities worksheet, 278
  aligning with present self, 276–277
  avoiding traps regarding, 264–266
  connecting with, 260–262
  Considering My True Nature worksheet, 263
  DBT Skills for Reaching My Future Self worksheet, 281–282
  former self and, 262–264
  identifying, 259–260
  Identifying My Current Behaviors worksheet, 262
  My Dangerous Driving Behaviors worksheet, 270
  My Dangerous Sexual Behaviors worksheet, 267–268
  My Drug and/or Alcohol Behaviors worksheet, 272–273
  My Future Me worksheet, 260
  My Future Qualities and Abilities worksheet, 279

G

Gratitude for the People No Longer in My Life worksheet, 237
grieving, inhibited, 223, 235–237
guilt, 137

H

Half-Smile, 197
harmful eating behaviors, 269
harmful short-term behaviors, 261
How Do I Know When I Am in My Wise Mind? worksheet, 114
How Fear Leads Me to Be Too Loose or Too Strict worksheet, 213–214
How my Emotions Are Impacted by Sleep Quality worksheet, 226
hypotheses about function of behavior, 97

I

I Am Fully Committed To... worksheet, 61
ice dive, 187
Identifying My Challenging Emotions and Associated Action Urges that Get Me Stuck worksheet, 150
Identifying My Current Behaviors worksheet, 262
identity narrative, 277
imagery, 183
Impact of Behavioral Dysregulation on My Life worksheet, 33

Impact of Cognitive Dysregulation on My Life worksheet, 37
Impact of Emotional Dysregulation on My Life worksheet, 30–31
Impact of Interpersonal Dysregulation On My Life worksheet, 35
Impact of Self-Dysregulation on My Life worksheet, 40
IMPROVE skill, 183–185
inhibited grieving, 223, 235–237
intense exercise, 187
intentional behavior
  breathing, 70–71
  choices
    rigid, 87–89
    value-driven, 91–93, 291–292
  letting go of attachment, 76–81
  My People worksheet, 75–76
  My Spaces worksheet, 73–74
  overview, 69–70
  perspective taking, 85–87
  Practicing Value-Driven Choices worksheet, 91–93
  relationships and
    overview, 72–76
    toxic, 82–84
  spaces and, 72–76
  Targeting My Attachment worksheet, 77–81
  Targeting My Point of View worksheet, 85–87
  Targeting Toxic Relationships worksheet, 82–84
  urge surfing, 71–72
  Walking the Middle Path, 90
interpersonal anger and conflict, managing with THINK skill, 173–177
interpersonal dysregulation, 9, 11, 33–35, 40
interpersonal effectiveness skills
  anger, managing with THINK skills, 173–177
  combining GIVE and FAST skills, 172–173
  DEAR MAN skills, 155–159
  FAST skills, 169–171
  GIVE skills, 167–169
  obstacles, 154–155
  overview, 153
  validation
    building blocks of, 161–163
    general discussion, 160–161
    practicing, 164–165
    self-validation, 161
    types of, 163
    when in disagreement, 165–166

invalidation, 23
It's Time to Use TIPP worksheet, 188

J

jealousy, 138
joy, 136
judgments, replacing with observable facts, 228
jumping to conclusions, 118
justified emotions, 139

L

lather rise repeat, 141
learning, continuous, 288
learning from emotions, 135
Learning from Past Emotional Decisions worksheet, 256–257
lifegoals, identifying, 56–57
Linehan, Marsha, 8–9
Losses I Have Experienced worksheet, 236
love, 136

M

Making a Choice worksheet, 67
Managing Interpersonal Anger and Conflict with the THINK Skill worksheet, 175–176
mastery, building, 294–295
meaning, 183
middle path
  dialectical dilemmas
    Assessing Typical Adolescent Behaviors worksheet, 216–217
    distinguishing problematic behaviors from typical behaviors, 215–216
    fostering dependency and forcing autonomy, 209–210
    How Fear Leads Me to Be Too Loose or Too Strict worksheet, 213–214
    too loose and too strict, 212–213
    Zooming In on Fostering Dependence and Forcing Autonomy worksheet, 210–212
  dialectical thinking, practicing, 205–208
  dialectics versus compromises, 204–205
  Generating Dialectical Thinking Using AND worksheet, 205–206
  overview, 203–208
  reacting with intention, 90
  Walking the Middle Path worksheet, 218–219

Miller, Alec, 203

mind reading, 118

mindfulness

  barriers to, 62

  benefits of, 110

  cognitive distortions, 118–119

  incorporating, 130–132

  of current thoughts, 116–117

  in distress tolerance model, 183

  emotion mind, 111–112

  How Do I Know When I Am in My Wise Mind? worksheet, 114

  "how" skills, 124–128

  Mindfulness of Current Thought Practices worksheet, 117

  My Emotion Mind Behaviors worksheet, 112

  My States of Mind worksheet, 115

  overview, 109–110

  practicing effectiveness, 129–130, 298

  problem-solving barriers to, 131–132

  Problem-Solving Barriers to My Mindfulness Practice worksheet, 131–132

  rational mind, 113–114

  states of mind, 111–115

  Times When I Need to Be in My Rational Mind worksheet, 113

  "what" skills, 120–124

  where and when of, 131

  Where and When of My Mindfulness Practice worksheet, 131

  wise mind, 113–115

  Working with My Cognitive Distortions worksheet, 119

money-spending behaviors, 271

mood-altering substances, avoiding, 142

mood-dependent behaviors

  as characteristics in BPD, 8

  cognitive distortions and, 87

  eliminating emotional decision making, 255–257

  emotional dysregulation and, 30

  goals and, 246–249

  Learning from Past Emotional Decisions worksheet, 256–257

  maintaining motivation, 250–253

  My Reflections on Obstacles worksheet, 254–255

  My Skills Plan for Warning Signs and Loss of Motivation worksheet, 252–253

  observing obstacles, 254–255

  regulating using DBT skills, 246

  Setting a Wise Goal worksheet, 247–248

  Signs I Am Losing Motivation worksheet, 252

  Taking My Goal from an Idea to Action worksheet, 249–250

motivation

  anticipating obstacles, 297

  encouraging patient to change, 24

  enhancing therapist's capabilities and, 25

  goals and, 56, 298

  maintaining, 250–253

  self-encouragement, 300

My Barriers to DBT Therapy worksheet, 63–64

My Barriers to Radical Acceptance worksheet, 194

My Crises Situations worksheet, 232–235

My Dangerous Driving Behaviors worksheet, 270

My Dangerous Sexual Behaviors worksheet, 267–268

My Drug and/or Alcohol Behaviors worksheet, 272–273

My Emotion Mind Behaviors worksheet, 112

My Experience of the Dialectical Dilemmas worksheet, 224

My Future Me worksheet, 260

My Future Qualities and Abilities worksheet, 279

My Goals worksheet, 286–288

My Harmful Eating Behaviors worksheet, 269

My Harmful Short-Term Behaviors worksheet, 261

My Identity Narrative worksheet, 277–278

My Lifegoals Are. . . worksheet, 56–57

My Money-Spending Behaviors worksheet, 271

My Negative Self-Talk and Negative Self-Judgments worksheet, 227–228

My People worksheet, 75–76

My Physical Reactions to Emotions worksheet, 225–226

My Problem Is. . . worksheet, 54–55

My Reasons for Engaging in Risky Behavior worksheet, 276

My Reflections on Obstacles worksheet, 254–255

My Self-Injury Behaviors worksheet, 273–274

My Skills Plan for Warning Signs and Loss of Motivation worksheet, 252–253

My Spaces worksheet, 73–74

My States of Mind worksheet, 115

My True Competencies worksheet, 230–232

My Wise Mind ACCEPTS worksheet, 182

N

naming emotions, 146
negative reinforcers, 99
negative self-talk and self-judgments, 227–228
news, limiting, 291–292

O

observable facts, replacing judgments with, 228
obstacles
  overcoming, 297–300
  reflecting on, 254–255
one thing in the moment skill, 183
opposite actions
  changing emotions with, 148–150
  practicing, 151–152
overgeneralization, 118

P

paced breathing, 187
paired muscle relaxation (PMR), 187
paradoxes, embracing, 238–241
past accomplishments, 66
past emotional decisions, learning from, 256–257
people in life, identifying emotions elicited by, 75–76
personalization, 118
physical reactions to emotions, 225–226
pivoting, 300
PLEASE Skills Red Flags and Reflection worksheet, 145
PMR (paired muscle relaxation), 187
point of view, targeting, 85–87
Positive and Negative Reinforcers worksheet, 99
Practicing Dialectical Thinking worksheet, 206–208
Practicing Effectiveness worksheet, 129–130
Practicing FAST Skills worksheet, 170–171
Practicing GIVE Skills worksheet, 168–169
Practicing My Pros and Cons worksheet, 192
Practicing Opposite Action worksheet, 151–152
Practicing Radical Acceptance worksheet, 195–196
Practicing the STOP Skill worksheet, 189–190
Practicing Validation worksheet, 164–165
Practicing Value-Driven Choices worksheet, 91–93
prayer, 183
present self, 276–282
primary emotions, 134–138

principle of impermanence, 264
problem areas in life, identifying, 47–49
problems
  assigning intention, avoiding, 50–51
  being specific about, 49–52
  in close relationships, 34–35
  controlling behaviors, 32
  dealing with emotions, 30
  defining, 46–47
  identifying, 43, 54–55
  solutions to, 44, 53–55, 299
  in thinking, 37
  understanding, 299
  vague language, avoiding, 49–50
pros and cons, listing, 190–192
psychological flexibility, 296
pushing away skill, 181

Q

qualities
  admiring in others, 278
  of future self, 279–280
Qualities I Need to Develop worksheet, 280–281
quality of sleep, 142, 226, 290–291

R

radical acceptance, 194–196
Rathus, Jill, 203
rational mind, 113
reactions
  first reaction, moving beyond
    attachment, letting go of, 76–81
    overview, 69–70
    sensing space, 72–76
    taking a breath, 70–71
    toxic relationships, letting go of, 82–84
    urge surfing, 71–72
  overview, 69
  reacting with intention
    overview, 85
    perspective taking, 85–87
    rigid choices, breaking free from, 87–93
reactivity, 8
red flags, PLEASE skills, 145

regulating emotions
  ABC PLEASE skill, 140–145
  benefits, 133–134
  overview, 139–140
  SUN WAVE NO NOT skill, 146–148
reinforcers, behavior, 98–99
relationships
  Answers worksheet, 177
  as barriers to commitment, 62
  DEAR MAN skill, 155–159
  Do I Have Problems in Close Relationships?
    worksheets, 34–35
  FAST skill, 169–173
  GIVE skill, 167–173
  Impact of Interpersonal Dysregulation On My Life
    worksheets, 35
  intentional behavior and, 72–76
  loneliness, 45
  Managing Interpersonal Anger and Conflict with the
    THINK Skill worksheet, 175–176
  My People worksheets, 75–76
  obstacles in, 154–155
  Practicing FAST Skills worksheet, 169–171
  Practicing GIVE Skills worksheet, 168–169
  Practicing Validation worksheet, 164–165
  social issues, 45
  Targeting Toxic Relationships worksheets, 82–84
  Things That Get in the Way of My Interpersonal
    Effectiveness worksheet, 155
  THINK skill, 173–177
  validation
    disagreements and, 165–167
    overview, 160–161
    types of, 161–167
  toxic, letting go of, 82–84
relaxation skills, 183
Replacing Judgments with Observable Facts worksheet,
  228
resignation, 194
risky behavior, reasons for engaging in, 276

S
sadness, 136, 140
SCREW acronym, 299
secondary emotions, 138–139
self-encouragement, 300

self-injury behaviors, 273–274
self-invalidation, 222, 226–228
self-soothing skills, 185–186
self-talk and self-judgments, negative, 227
self-validation
  benefits of, 301–302
  steps for, 302–308
  understanding one's emotions, 161
sensations, 182
sense of self, 10, 38–40. See also future self
sense-of-self dysregulation, 10, 12, 38–40
Setting a Wise Goal worksheet, 247–248
sexual behaviors, dangerous, 267–268
shame, 137
shaping behaviors, 104
Shaping Behaviors worksheet, 104
short- and long-term goals, clarifying, 58–59
short-term behaviors, harmful, 261
sleep quality, 142, 226, 290–291
social media, limiting use of, 291–292

T
temperature, 187
thoughts skill, 181–182
TIPP skill, 187–188
toxic relationships, targeting, 82–84
true nature, considering, 263
"turning the mind" skill, 196–197

U
unjustified emotions, 139
unrelenting crises, 223, 232–235
urges
  identifying, 150
  SUN WAVE NO NOT method, 146
  urge surfing, 71–72

V
vacation skill, 183
validation
  disagreements and, 165–167
  emotions, 298
  overview, 160–161

practicing, 164–165

self-validation

benefits of, 301–302

steps for, 302–308

understanding one's emotions with, 161

types of, 161–166

Validation and Invalidation worksheet, 22–23

value-driven choices, practicing, 91–93

visualizing future self, 265–266

Visualizing My Future Self worksheet, 265–266

W

Walking the Middle Path

Assessing Typical Adolescent Behaviors worksheet, 216–217

dialectics versus compromises, 204–205

fostering dependency and forcing autonomy, 209–210

Generating Dialectical Thinking Using AND worksheet, 205–206

How Fear Leads Me to Be Too Loose or Too Strict worksheet, 213–214

overview, 203–208

Practicing Dialectical Thinking worksheet, 206–208

problematic versus typical adolescent behaviors, 215–216

reacting with intention, 90

too loose and too strict, 212–213

Walking the Middle Path worksheet, 218–219

Zooming In on Fostering Dependence and Forcing Autonomy worksheet, 210–212

warning signs, skills plan for, 252–253

WAVE, riding the, 146

Ways to Embrace My Paradoxes worksheet, 241

weekly tracking of ABC PLEASE skills, 144–145

What I Learned from My Emotions worksheet, 135

Where and When of My Mindfulness Practice worksheet, 131

wholistic health, practicing, 288–291

willfulness, 197–199

Willing Hands, 197

willingness, 197–199

wise goals, setting, 247–248

wise mind, 113–115

Wise Mind ACCEPTS skill, 182

Working with My Cognitive Distortions worksheet, 119

About the Authors

Gillian Galen, PsyD, is an instructor of psychology at Harvard Medical School and the Director of Training for the 3East DBT Continuum of Care at McLean Hospital in Belmont, Massachusetts. Gillian has extensive experience diagnosing and treating adolescents and young adults who struggle with emotion dysregulation, anxiety, depression, trauma, and self-endangering behaviors, such as self-injury and suicidal behaviors. She has a particular interest in working with and supporting families who have loved ones who struggle with these behaviors and symptoms. Gillian is the co-author of *DBT for Dummies, Mindfulness for Borderline Personality Disorder,* and *Coping With BPD.*

Blaise Aguirre, MD, is the Founding Medical Director of 3East, a DBT continuum of care at McLean Hospital in Belmont, Massachusetts, and a trainer in dialectical behavior therapy. Blaise is an assistant professor of psychiatry at Harvard Medical School. He has been a staff psychiatrist at McLean Hospital since 2000 and is nationally and internationally recognized for his extensive work in the treatment of mood and personality disorders in adolescents. He lectures regularly throughout the world. Blaise is the author or co-author of many books, including: *Borderline Personality Disorder in Adolescents, Mindfulness for Borderline Personality Disorder,* and *Coping With BPD.*

Dedication

This book is dedicated to anyone who yearns for a more skillful life and for the people who courageously face the pain in their lives and persist despite obstacles. We also dedicate this book to Marsha Linehan, the developer of DBT, our teachers, and every DBT colleague committed to helping those who ask for their help.

Authors' Acknowledgments

We want to recognize our DBT team at McLean Hospital as well as our private practice DBT team. They make sure that we stay committed to the work and dedicated to the principles and protocols of DBT.

We deeply appreciate our team at Wiley — Tracy Boggier, who patiently waited until we were ready to write this book, and Kezia Endsley, who helped shape the contents.

To all our past and present clients. You have been the inspiration that showed us the power of DBT. Thank you for allowing us to be companions on your journey and trusting us to guide you.

To our dear friend and colleague, Dr. Anna Precht, PhD, who made sure that the content was accurate.

And finally, to our loudest cheerleader, Mika Brzezinski, who embodies the practice and power of DBT.

Publisher's Acknowledgments

Acquisitions Editor: Tracy Boggier

Editorial Project Manager and Editor: Kezia Endsley

Technical Editor: Dr. Anna Precht, PhD

Production Editor: Tamilmani Varadharaj

Cover Image: © Romolo Tavani/Shutterstock

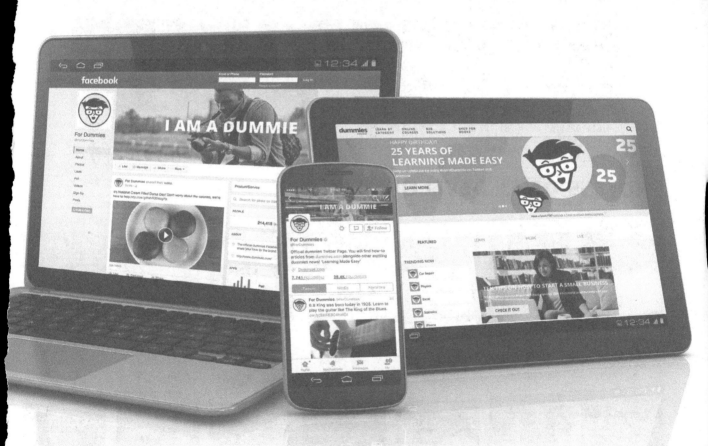

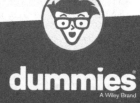

PERSONAL ENRICHMENT

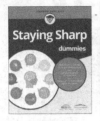
9781119187790
USA $26.00
CAN $31.99
UK £19.99

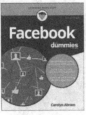
9781119179030
USA $21.99
CAN $25.99
UK £16.99

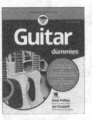
9781119293354
USA $24.99
CAN $29.99
UK £17.99

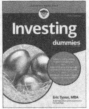
9781119293347
USA $22.99
CAN $27.99
UK £16.99

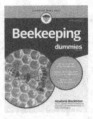
9781119310068
USA $22.99
CAN $27.99
UK £16.99

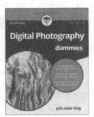
9781119235606
USA $24.99
CAN $29.99
UK £17.99

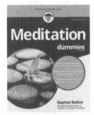
9781119251163
USA $24.99
CAN $29.99
UK £17.99

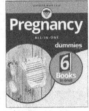
9781119235491
USA $26.99
CAN $31.99
UK £19.99

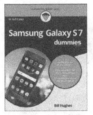
9781119279952
USA $24.99
CAN $29.99
UK £17.99

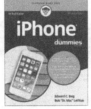
9781119283133
USA $24.99
CAN $29.99
UK £17.99

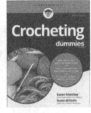
9781119287117
USA $24.99
CAN $29.99
UK £16.99

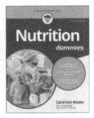
9781119130246
USA $22.99
CAN $27.99
UK £16.99

PROFESSIONAL DEVELOPMENT

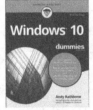
9781119311041
USA $24.99
CAN $29.99
UK £17.99

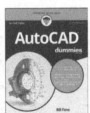
9781119255796
USA $39.99
CAN $47.99
UK £27.99

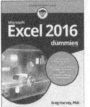
9781119293439
USA $26.99
CAN $31.99
UK £19.99

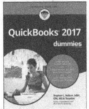
9781119281467
USA $26.99
CAN $31.99
UK £19.99

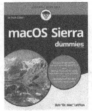
9781119280651
USA $29.99
CAN $35.99
UK £21.99

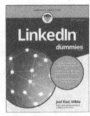
9781119251132
USA $24.99
CAN $29.99
UK £17.99

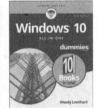
9781119310563
USA $34.00
CAN $41.99
UK £24.99

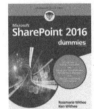
9781119181705
USA $29.99
CAN $35.99
UK £21.99

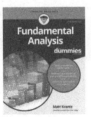
9781119263593
USA $26.99
CAN $31.99
UK £19.99

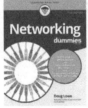
9781119257769
USA $29.99
CAN $35.99
UK £21.99

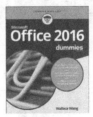
9781119293477
USA $26.99
CAN $31.99
UK £19.99

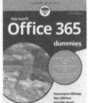
9781119265313
USA $24.99
CAN $29.99
UK £17.99

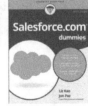
9781119239314
USA $29.99
CAN $35.99
UK £21.99

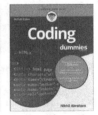
9781119293323
USA $29.99
CAN $35.99
UK £21.99

dummies.com

dummies
A Wiley Brand